G000256311

Soccer Injuries

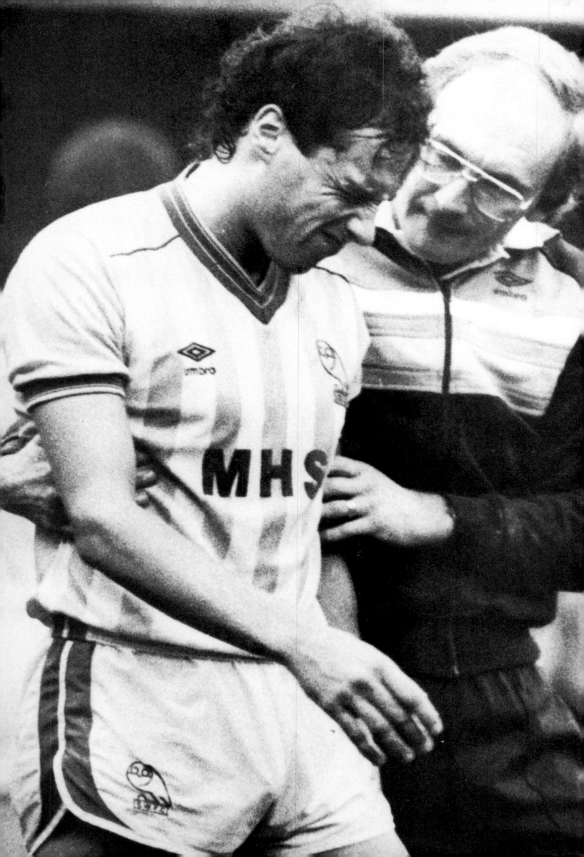

SOCCER INJURIES
PREVENTION AND FIRST AID

ALAN G. SMITH
MCSP, LCSP(Phys)

The Crowood Press

First published in 1989 by
The Crowood Press
Ramsbury, Marlborough,
Wiltshire SN8 2HE

© Alan G. Smith 1989

All rights reserved. No part of this publication may be reproduced or
transmitted in any form or by any means, electronic or mechanical,
including photocopy, recording, or any information storage and
retrieval system without permission in writing from the publishers.

British Library Cataloguing in Publication Data
Smith, Alan
    Soccer injuries, prevention and first aid
    1.   Association footballers.   Injuries
    I.   Title
    617'.1027

    ISBN 1–85223–186–6

**Dedicated to my wife Judith for her help and
kindness in typing my words and to my sons Paul
and Andrew for their understanding during
the preparation of this book.**

Acknowledgements
All photographs by Steve Ellis except
Fig 20 courtesy of the *Blackpool Gazette & Herald*
and Fig 77 courtesy of the *Sunderland Echo*.
Cover photographs by Steve Ellis.
Cover design by Vic Giolitto.

Typeset by Columns of Reading
Printed in Great Britain by Redwood Burn Ltd, Trowbridge

Contents

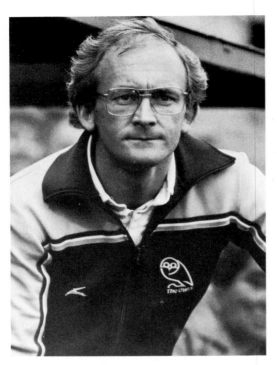

Alan G. Smith, MCSP, LCSP (Phys), is physiotherapist for Sheffield Wednesday FC and the England Under-21 team.

This book will be a great help to the many thousands of people responsible for the first-aid treatment of soccer injuries. I feel that it will educate and prepare you to deal with the injured footballer correctly.

Bobby Robson
England Team Manager

I have had twenty-seven years as a coach and manager at all levels. I have worked with Alan for the past eight years with the England Under-21 team and I can guarantee that this book will be of benefit both to those who administer treatment and more importantly those who suffer injuries in the course of our great game, football.

Dave Sexton
England Under-21 Team Manager

This book is excellent value. Alan gives a highly valued opinion on the principles of soccer injury management and initial treatment procedures.

Alan Ball
Former England captain

Referees at all levels of the game should read this book. Alan's comments will assist them in their decision-making in regard to players' injuries.

Keith Hackett
FIFA referee

A superb physio whose undivided attention from minute one till eighteen months later has almost certainly saved my leg and with it my footballing career.
  A man of unequalled and outstanding knowledge of his profession. Top class!

Ian Knight
Sheffield Wednesday FC

Foreword

Several years ago, when we started the sports injuries clinic at the Northern General Hospital in Sheffield, a young man joined us as an accredited observer. His interest and enthusiasm was impressive, and it was clear that his aim was to become a sports physiotherapist.

That young man is the author of this book. It was no surprise to those of us who knew him to hear that he had realised his ambition and had become a member of the Chartered Society of Physiotherapy, that he had become physiotherapist to a very well-known soccer club and finally that he had attained the ultimate honour of being appointed by the Football Association as a member of the physiotherapy staff to serve the England international teams.

It has long been his wish to write an instruction manual – summarising his considerable experience at home and abroad – mainly for the very large number of 'trainers' with the host of local league, youth and schoolboy teams who give their services voluntarily because of their love of sport, but who for various reasons have had no opportunity to gain specialised teaching and training in physiotherapy.

This manual is the result of his endeavours. It is written in clear and simple terms, stressing the supreme importance of basic principles of therapy and advising on essential basic equipment. It is illustrated with excellent diagrams and pictures supporting the text, which is a summary of his own considerable experience in the management of all types of injury in sport. When it is essential for an understanding of the injury, he has described the anatomy in simple terms, but he has deliberately avoided comment on the very specialised topics of biochemistry and psychology.

This book should have a wide appeal to all involved in sport; participants, coaches and physiotherapists. I wish it every success.

Frank O'Gorman *MRCP, FRCS, FRCOG*
Emeritus Professor of Surgery
University of Sheffield
Honorary Consultant Physician, FA
Medical Adviser, FIFA

Preface

This book is dedicated to the many thousands of people who freely give their spare time to organise football throughout the country. Without their enthusiasm and dedication the game would not prosper and it is for these people that I decided to write this book, my aim being to produce a book that is easily understood yet informative. I have based the information on injuries received on the field of play, and also include discussion of the mechanics of injury, signs and symptoms, initial management, first-aid treatment and the principles of treatment.

Every football club should have a person specifically appointed to treat injuries. That individual ought to be encouraged to attend a first-aid course run by an organisation such as the St John Ambulance or the British Red Cross Society. Alternatively, since 1949 the Football Association have held an excellent annual course on the treatment of injuries at Lilleshall (the coaching regions also organise courses locally). For further details on these courses, write to the Football Association (*see* Useful Addresses).

1 Prevention of Injury

The prevention of injury to members of your football club is naturally of major importance and their well-being the responsibility of the club that they represent. As an official for the team, you should make an effort to educate your players in the ways in which the incidence of injury can be reduced and avoidable injury prevented. The following principles ought to be observed and acted upon by all players.

FOOT CARE

To prepare your feet against blisters, bathe them during the pre-season period in potassium permanganate. This should be applied in a foot bowl with tepid water to a depth of about 5cm (2in), in which a pinch of potassium permanganate has been dissolved. After showering, stand in the bowl for thirty seconds and then dry your feet thoroughly. Apply surgical spirit with the aid of cotton-wool balls to those areas of the feet most vulnerable to blisters. (Do not apply surgical spirit to an open blister.)

Apply Vaseline or white petroleum jelly to your stocking toes and heels in order to reduce friction and introduce new footwear gradually – do not leave it until your existing pair of training shoes or boots has worn out. Buy a new pair a little in advance and wear them in gradually so that you are not suddenly left with uncomfortable foot-wear – this is particularly important during the pre-season period.

Fungal infections such as athlete's foot are very common irritants. Prior to the start of pre-season training, educate your players to dry thoroughly both between the toes (and around the groin); after drying dust with a suitable powder. Also, wearing flip flops in the dressing-room, bathroom and shower areas can prevent the spreading of fungal problems, verrucae as well as reduce the risk of blisters becoming infected.

The cutting of toe nails, although sounding insignificant, is something players ought to do regularly and correctly. Poorly cut nails can give rise to problems particularly ingrowing toe nails, which could lead to a player missing matches. The preventative measure in this instance is to cut the nail square and file the edges and corners.

WARMING UP

Before each training session or game, a warming up routine should be performed by all the players who are to take an active part in the proceedings. Use a progressive system of jogging, skipping, running (with high knee action and high heel lift), side jogging, back pedalling and running sequences increasing speed. The aim here is to raise the pulse rate gradually. In doing this the blood supply to the muscles is increased and once a

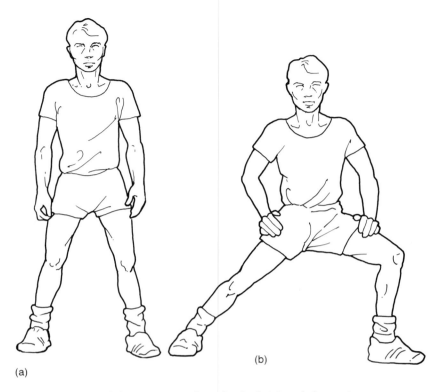

(a)

(b)

Fig 1 *Starting position of the groin stretch, right thigh (a) and the position showing the extensibility of the right adductor complex (groin) (b).*

pulse rate of approximately 120 beats per minute is reached then the muscle groups that will be used in the course of the game (these include the groin, hamstring, quadriceps and calf) can be stretched. (*See* Figs 1–4.)

For the dressing-room warm-up, oil of wintergreen or similar rubs are of little value. The best and correct way to prepare is to follow an exercise routine within the dressing-room area if the weather conditions or circumstances do not allow you to work outside. The exercise routine might be as follows:

1. Running on the spot.
2. Step-ups on to a bench.
3. Half-squats to a bench.
4. Alternate toe touching.
5. Sprinting on the spot.

Once the pulse has reached 120 beats per minute, stop and stretch the muscle groups mentioned above.

RECOVERY AND MAINTAINING FITNESS

Great care must be taken to ensure that your players do not return to the game too soon after a bout of flu or viral infection. A consultation and examination by your doctor should be carried

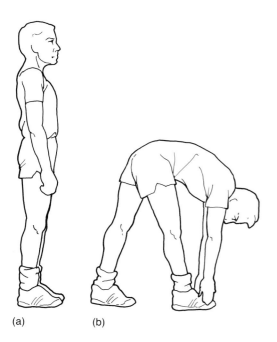

Fig 2 Starting position of the hamstring stretch, right thigh (a) and the position showing the extensibility of the hamstring muscle group of the forward position leg (b).

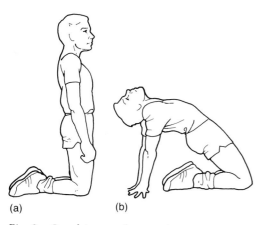

Fig 3 Quadriceps: the starting position (a) and the position showing the stretching ability of the rectus femoris of both thighs (b).

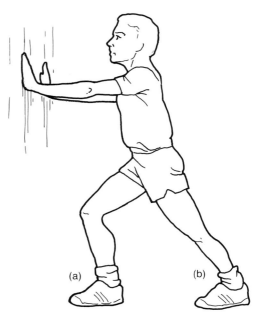

Fig 4 Calf: the stretching of the gastro-cnemius and soleus (a) and the stretching of the calf muscle group (b).

out before the player returns to the team. Maintaining fitness during the close season is of importance. Playing tennis, swimming, jogging or even cricket will help to retain a degree of fitness. To give the players a moderate exercise programme at the end of the season is another method that can be adopted. Progressive jogging and distance running can be geared towards the beginning of pre-season training.

OTHER PRECAUTIONS

Hygiene is also important; clean dressing-rooms, baths and shower areas should be a priority and each individual using only his own towel is a commonsense

11

procedure. In addition, he should use his own kit for training and not borrow from a team-mate.

Vaccination against tetanus ought to be a club rule: a record should be kept of each individual once he is immunised. Your doctor can also help to protect the players against the risk of contracting poliomyelitis and flu, if he thinks it necessary.

An examination of the area you are about to train or play on can be of value in avoiding injury. A poor, uneven surface can lead to injury and should, of course, be avoided if possible.

Wearing the correct footwear for the type of surface you are about to play on is important, particularly so for younger, inexperienced players who should perhaps be educated to know when to wear a moulded, studded boot rather than a boot with long or short studs. Additionally, the wearing of shin pads for all games should be a club rule, as should the banning of signet-rings, chewing-gum – and dentures! – during a match.

FITNESS

Football demands both skill and fitness and one major contribution to reducing the risk of injury is to possess a high degree of physical fitness. The aims of physical fitness, so far as injury prevention is concerned, are roughly as follows:

1. *Endurance* The main physiological aims are to reduce the onset of fatigue by improving the efficiency of heart, lungs and circulatory systems. The benefits of achieving this are great since tired players make mistakes and a player suffering from fatigue will work

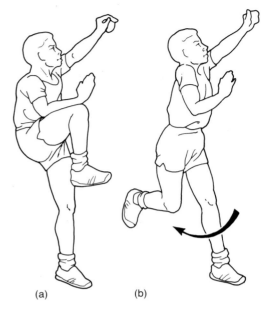

(a) (b)

Fig 5 Hip flexion (a) and extension (b).

less efficiently and be susceptible to making errors in judgement. These factors make the individual prone to injury.

A good method of improving your players' endurance is to devise a progressive series of cross-country running courses and incorporate these into your training programme. You might wish to add some circuit-training which involves a low weight-resistance but a high number of repetitions.

2. *Mobility* During the course of a game a player's joints may well be stretched to the extreme end of their normal mobility range or a muscle group pulled to the limit of its extensibility. A clinical limitation of a joint's range of movement could contribute to injury. Extensibility exercises are described in this chapter and Figs 5–7 illustrate how to determine the range of mobility of a particular joint.

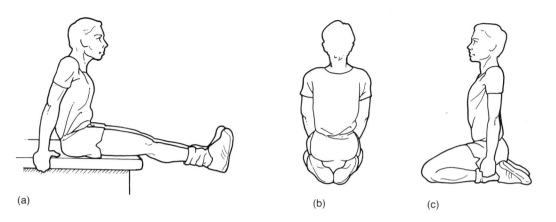

(a) (b) (c)

Fig 6   *The knee joint, extension (a) and flexion, rear view (b), side view (c).*

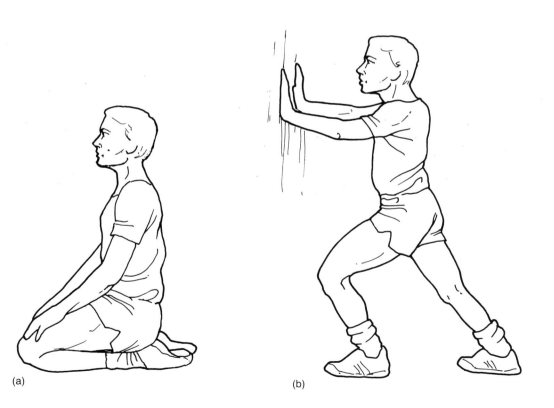

(a) (b)

Fig 7   *The ankle joint, plantar flexion (a) and dorsiflexion (b).*

13

3. *Strength* To improve your players' strength, a programme of lifting should be devised with a high weight-resistance and a low number of repetitions and sprints in the form of shuttle-runs over short distances (perhaps 20m or 22 yds). The instruction to your players should be to incorporate explosive power into their sprinting effort.

4. *Skill* Poor techniques when tackling, controlling the ball, shooting, crossing or passing can occasionally lead to an injury. Repetitive practice is the only way to improve and so reduce this (minor) risk of injury.

2 Treatment on the Field of Play

When dealing with injuries on the field it is important to follow the following rules of procedure:

1. If you actually observe the incident in which the injury was sustained, do not be tempted to pre-diagnose. Always approach an injury with 'an open mind'.
2. On reaching the player on the field, ask him how the injury occurred; was it the result of a direct blow or perhaps a twist?
3. Ask for active movement of the limb, never apply passive movement.
4. Apply your treatment once a diagnosis has been established.
5. When in doubt remove the player from the field and seek professional medical advice.
6. In the case of a lower limb, back or spinal injury, do not allow the player to stand before examination and diagnosis have been completed.

LIGAMENT INJURIES

For footballers the medial ligament (inside) of the knee joint and the lateral ligament (outside) of the ankle joint are the two main areas for ligamentous injury. The usual medial ligament injury involves the knee joint being forced into a valgus or knock-kneed position, so stretching the tissue. The usual lateral ligament injury involves the ankle joint being forced into plantar flexion and inversion – commonly known as 'going over' on the ankle. When treating both types of injury, the following points, with regard to severity, symptoms and initial management, should be borne in mind:

1. *The mild sprain* The active function is full, but a little painful; no effusion (swelling). Apply cold water or pain-relief spray and allow the player to continue the game.
2. *The moderate sprain* A number of ligament fibres have been torn, resulting in a very painful injury with associated limitation of active movement. There is an immediate, moderate effusion and you may be able to detect a slight rise in temperature – evident from palpations – over the site of injury. The player so injured is unable to continue the game.
3. *The severe injury* The most severe degree of isolated injury to ligamentous tissue is the complete rupture. The force of the injury is quite considerable and produces the most extreme symptoms; an immediate effusion with associated temperature rise in the joint. The pain is excruciating and the player may believe he has a fracture. There is also a gross loss of active movement. This injury should be immobilised as though it were a fracture and the player taken from the

field on a stretcher and transported to hospital.

THE OPEN WOUND

Minor wounds should be thoroughly cleaned with Cetavlon 1% dabbed on to a piece of gauze or cotton wool and then protected by a sterile dressing. If you are uncertain about the seriousness of a particular injury, remove the player from the field so that a more detailed examination may be carried out. Severe wounds that require suturing must be treated as quickly as possible. Clean the wound, apply a dressing and arrange for transport to hospital. If a wound is bleeding profusely, apply pressure to the wound and to the nearest arterial anatomical pressure point and transport the casualty to the hospital.

THE RIB FRACTURE

This will have been caused by a direct blow to the rib cage. An undisplaced fracture will cause the player to take shallow breaths, minimising any disturbance of the fracture and reducing the pain. However, inhalation will be very

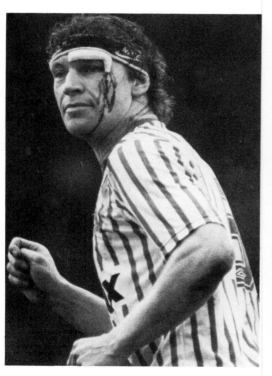

Fig 8   Ian Cranson, centre-half for Sheffield Wednesday, pictured after suffering a head-wound.

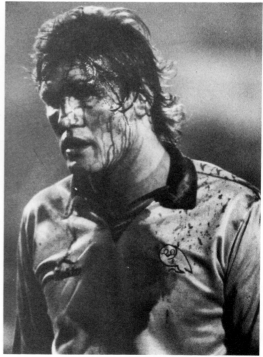

Fig 9   Mike Lyons of Sheffield Wednesday leaving the field for treatment to a head-wound.

uncomfortable and a player showing these symptoms should be removed from the field and referred to hospital. When a player suffers more than one fracture with a degree of displacement, the symptoms are the same but more pronounced. The player should be stretchered from the field with his body positioned so that the site of injury is tilted downwards.

INJURY TO THE FACE

Fractures of the nasal bone are the most common of all facial fractures and should be taken seriously since impaired respiratory problems can result from an untreated displacement. An examination for concussion should be carried out as well as an X-ray of the nasal bone. Players also suffer from the occasional nose bleed following minor knocks and when trying to stop the bleeding the best technique is to apply internal and external pressure; place a piece of cotton wool soaked in Vaseline into the nostril (or nostrils) and apply pressure by holding the soft part of the nose between finger and thumb for a few minutes.

Fractures to the upper and lower jaw are infrequent, but if you are presented with a lower-jaw fracture you will find that the player will be unable to control his saliva (probably blood-stained) and will have difficulty in speaking. The treatment is to support the jaw with a triangular bandage, ensure the player is able to breathe adequately and remove him from the field on a stretcher (in the recovery position), then arrange transport to hospital.

CRAMP

Cramp is a very painful and sometimes long-lasting spasm or contraction of a muscle or muscle group. It is caused, ultimately, by a lack of fitness. The wearing of 'tie-ups' that restrict the circulation and playing in the extreme temperatures may also cause cramp. The treatment is to stretch the affected muscle group with passive assistance (that is you, and not the player, work the muscle backwards and forwards) until the spasm has cleared.

THE TESTICLES AND SCROTUM

A direct blow to the scrotal region produces an extremely painful injury. If the pain does not pass quickly, take the player off the field and seek medical advice. The best treatment for the relief of pain is the direct application of warm water. The procedure for diagnosing more serious injury is to examine the player's urine for any traces of blood. If blood is present you must inform the player's doctor or casualty staff on arrival at hospital.

FRACTURES

The most common cause of a fractured bone is a direct blow, but occasionally you may find that a rotational stress to the leg, when supporting the full weight, will produce a fracture, as will 'indirect violence'; for example a blow to the inside of the ankle, forcing the player to go over on the ankle, may cause a fracture to the fibula on the side opposite to the contact. The obvious symptoms include considerable pain and a lack of active movement, as well as swelling and deformity. For a less severe fracture the symptoms are less pronounced; diminished active movement, pain and local swelling.

The first-aid treatment on the field must immobilise the fracture either by the application of an inflatable splint or by moving the sound leg to the fractured leg and tying the legs firmly together with triangular bandages. These techniques will be more fully described in Chapter 4.

HEAD INJURIES

In football the two main injuries to the head are either damage to brain tissue or a fracture of the skull. These conditions can arise from a clash of heads, a kick or a blow from an elbow.

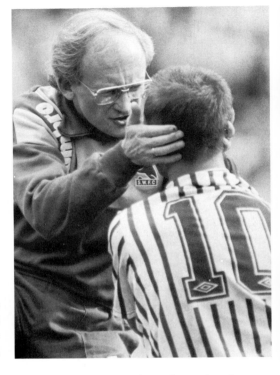

Fig 10 An examination of a player's pupils following a head injury.

Concussion

The symptoms are evident; the player will be unaware of the incident, dull and listless. Your examination should first check for a head-wound then study the pupils to observe their reaction to light. Place your hands over the player's closed eyes for about thirty seconds, then remove your hands and ask the player to open his eyes. The pupils of the eyes will have dilated (become larger) while covered by your hands and on exposure to light should constrict (become smaller), providing the player is not suffering from a concussion. If the player's pupils respond fairly quickly, this will give you a good indication that the player will soon recover and be able to continue the game. However, if on exposure to light the pupils do not constrict the player should be taken off the field and professional medical advice sought. You should also ask some simple questions to test the player's mental ability, such as the score or the name of the opposition.

Unconsciousness

If a player is unconscious, you must first ensure that he has an airway by placing him in the recovery position (*see* Fig 13) and then check his heart is still beating by placing your finger over the carotid artery at the side of the neck. Because

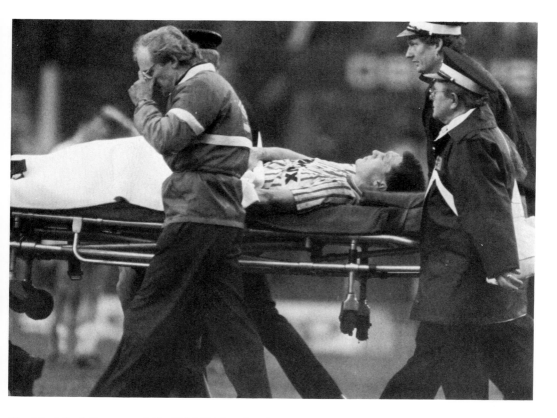

Fig 11   Nigel Pearson of Sheffield Wednesday being stretchered off at Old Trafford after suffering a fracture and dislocation of his left ankle.

the player has been taking strenuous exercise, his pulse can easily be detected. The player should be taken from the field on a stretcher, still in the recovery position and then to hospital by ambulance.

If the player has swallowed his tongue, place him in the recovery position, ensuring full extension of the neck which should remove the blockage by the tongue. (If he has stopped breathing, immediately start resuscitation using the mouth-to-mouth method, *see* below.) Check that he has a good airway, support the nape of the neck and gently press the top of the head so that it is tilted backwards, pushing the chin upwards. This extends the head and neck and lifts the tongue forward, clear of the airway. If the player is capable of breathing this may be the only move necessary, and he will gasp and start to breathe. At this point place him in the recovery position.

RESUSCITATION

If the player does not respond the following procedure is recommended:

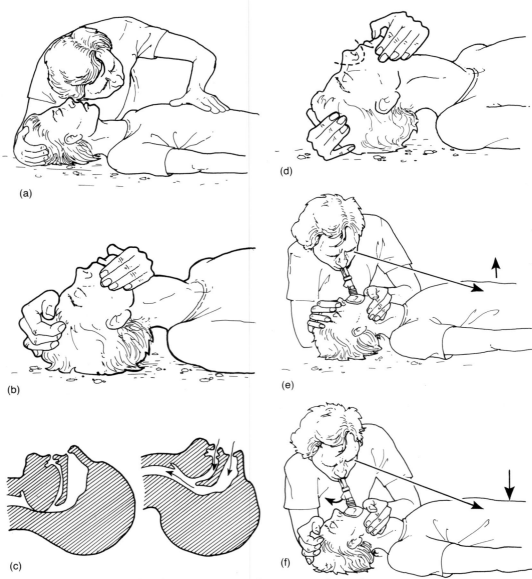

Fig 12 *The procedure for the resuscitation of an unconscious player. First, check for breathing by placing your hand on the player's chest and by moving your face close to his mouth and nose to feel and hear any breathing (a). Then position the casualty's head correctly so that the airway is free of obstruction (b and c). Next compress the nostrils (d) and with your left hand gently open the player's mouth, placing the Brook airway in position. Then breathe through the airway so that the player's chest is seen to rise (e) and fall (f).*

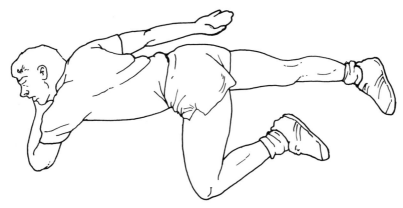

Fig 13   The recovery position.

1.   Lay the player flat on his back and tilt his chin up so that his neck is not constricted. To check for respiration put your ear to his mouth and listen (and feel) for breathing; you may also place your hand on his chest to detect any rise and fall.

2.   Clear the player's mouth and check that the airway is clear – chewing-gum must be forbidden during training and competitive play.

3.   Place the resuscitator in the player's mouth.

4.   Open your mouth and take a deep breath.

5.   Pinch the casualty's nostrils together between your thumb and index finger.

6.   Seal your lips around the resuscitator.

7.   Blow until the player's chest rises.

8.   Remove your mouth and watch the chest fall.

9.   Repeat inflations at a normal rate of breathing.

EXTERNAL HEART COMPRESSION

When you cannot feel the carotid pulse, you should then use external heart compression as follows:

1.   Position yourself to the side of the player.

2.   Feel for the lowest part of the sternum (breastbone). Position the heel of your right hand slightly to the (player's) left of the sternum.

3.   Cover your right hand with your left.

4.   With your arms straight, push forwards pressing down on to the lower part of the sternum and ribs directly over the heart.

5.   The compression should be repeated at a rate of five compressions for two quick lung inflations. This ratio should be repeated continuously until the pulse can be felt and breathing starts again.

6.   Once breathing has recommenced place the player in the recovery position.

7.   Arrange for an ambulance to take the player to hospital.

21

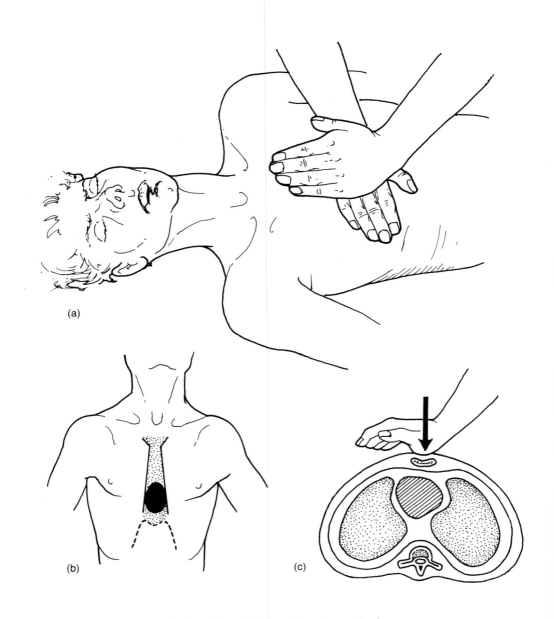

(a)

(b)

(c)

Fig 14   *Cardiac massage: the hand should be positioned over the lower part of the sternum and the heart (a); the position on the sternum where pressure should be applied (b); the position of the heel of the hand shown in relation to the sternum and the heart (c).*

THE USE OF STRETCHERS

Having immobilised or correctly positioned a seriously injured player, a stretcher is then required to carry him from the field. You can choose to place the stretcher in one of two positions; by the side or at the feet of the injured player. If you choose the first of these two options, you are of course restricted to lifting him from only one side of his body, since there should be no one between the player and the stretcher. Moreover, those lifting the player must take one or possibly two steps before laying the player on the stretcher.

If the stretcher is positioned at the feet of the injured player, he may then be lifted from both sides. In this situation, it is essential that you take charge of the proceedings and ensure that helpers are positioned adequately to lift the player safely. After you have counted 'one, two, three, lift', the casualty should be raised roughly two feet in the air and the stretcher slid under the full length of his body. Delegate a person to each of the four corners of the stretcher and tell them to prepare themselves to lift and carry the stretcher at the instruction of 'one, two, three, lift'. Walk off the pitch taking the shortest route to the dressing-room area or waiting ambulance.

3 The Principles of Treatment

DIAGNOSIS

Diagnosis must always be the first priority with an injury, for if you fail to diagnose an injury correctly then your treatment will almost certainly fail. Professional medical advice should be sought if possible, and always if you are uncertain of the diagnosis.

THE ACUTE STAGE

Ice should be applied to all soft tissue injuries for a period of ten to fifteen minutes. For this application you can use a chemical ice-pack, ice-cubes placed into a plastic bag or crushed ice – whichever you choose, it should be stored in an ice bucket and kept, ready for use, in the dressing-room. When using ice, you should always protect the skin from possible burns by applying olive oil or a plastic bag between the site of injury and the ice. Heat of any kind should be kept away from the injury during the acute stage, and your players educated to shower quickly rather than take a bath following a game if they have an injury. (The application of ice not only reduces pain but also minimises swelling by constricting the blood vessels so stopping any bleeding.)

COMPRESSION

The application of pressure to a soft tissue injury is of vital importance, but techniques differ according to which part of the anatomy is injured although the principles remain the same: to prevent the injured tissue from being damaged further, you should immobilise it, and secondly to apply a pressure bandage, which will spread the resulting inflammatory exudate following injury and help to reduce pain.

REST

A rest period of between twenty-four and forty-eight hours is recommended depending on the severity of injury. By resting, the player's pulse rate will decrease – desirable in the initial stage of injury management when bleeding may continue – and obviously the resting period will prevent any disturbance of the injured tissues.

ELEVATION

Whenever possible, it is advisable to elevate an injured area (as well as adopting those measures mentioned earlier): the player should lie with the limb supported on pillows so that the site of injury is above the rest of the body. This procedure will allow inflammatory

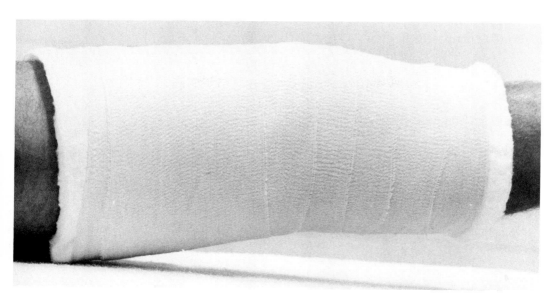

Fig 15   *The complete pressure bandage for the knee joint.*

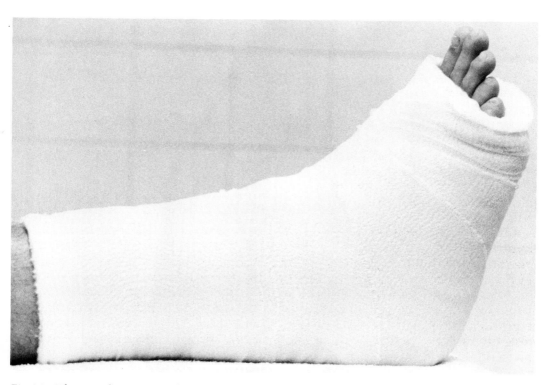

Fig 16   *The complete pressure bandage for a second degree sprain of the
ankle ligaments.*

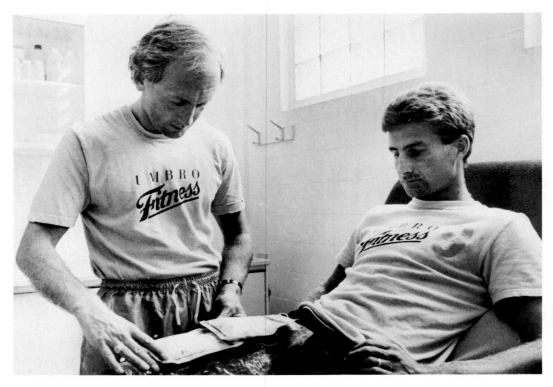

Fig 17   The application of ice to a thigh injury, using two chemical ice-packs. Note the protective layer between the ice and the skin (a plastic bag is also quite sufficient).

exudate to be asborbed into the lymphatic and venous systems, reduce tissue pressure and so decrease pain.

TISSUE REACTION TO INJURY

When a player receives an injury, irrespective of what structure is damaged, blood vessels are ruptured, giving rise to the trauma of plasma, blood cells, platelets and, in the case of fractures, bone cells passing into the surrounding tissue. These initial reactions create the following inflammatory symptoms: temperature; redness; pain; swelling and reduced active function.

TISSUE REPAIR FOLLOWING INJURY

Firstly, a blood clot is formed by blood platelets. Next, the white corpuscles clear the area of the dead tissue and the blood clot, so allowing the development of capillary buds, which grow across the injured area. These buds gradually meet and form capillaries, allowing the red corpuscles to establish a new circulation. Fibroblasts then begin to lay down fibrils, from which collagen is formed. This, basically, is the fibrous tissue of repair.

4 Fractures

Fractures may be caused by direct or indirect violence, by fatigue (stress fracture) or by disease (pathological fracture). A fracture may be either closed (simple) or compound (when the skin has been broken by either the fractured bone or as the result of direct contact by a player's boot or stud).

DIRECT VIOLENCE

Direct violence is said to be the cause of a fracture when the bone breaks at or near the site of violence. The type of fracture depends on the amount of force applied, the angle at which contact is made, the type of associated joints and the age of the player concerned. For example an accidental kick on the shin may give rise to a transverse fracture of the tibia without displacement whereas a violent blow may bend the bone and cause angulation at the site of the fracture.

INDIRECT VIOLENCE

Indirect violence is said to be the cause when force is applied at a point or points other than the site of the fracture. The position and type of fracture may depend upon the position of the bone at the time of receiving the injury; fractures of the upper limb can be received by falling on to an outstretched hand resulting in a fractured scaphoid or a Colles fracture of the wrist. If the force producing the fracture is rotational, a spiral fracture may be found in either the fibula or tibia in the leg and the radius or ulna in the arm. It is not common to sustain a fracture of the clavicle by falling on an out-stretched hand or arm.

TYPES OF FRACTURE

Greenstick This fracture is associated with childhood and involves the bone bending on one side and fracturing on the opposite side.

Transverse This type of break occurs when a transverse line of fracture is visible across the bone.

Angulated This is when a triangular fragment or fragments are split from the concave side of the fracture.

Oblique or Spiral The bone will have been rotated or twisted along its long axis to produce this type of fracture.

Comminuted This type of fracture is caused by direct violence and results in a jigsaw of fractures within the bone.

Joint Fracture The fracture line extends into and through the articular cartilage of a joint.

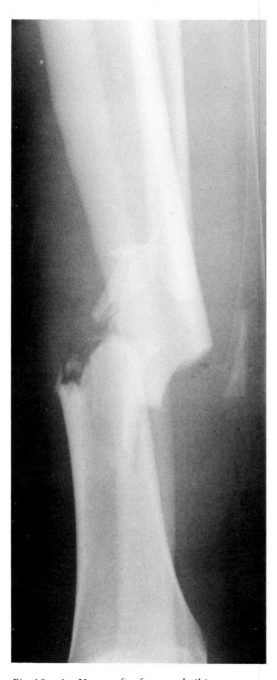

Fig 18   An X-ray of a fractured tibia.

Avulsion The force applied to the ligament detaches a flake of bone.

Fracture Dislocation This is when a fracture is associated with a dislocated joint or the position of the fracture makes the joint unstable. The Pott's fracture of the ankle is the most common fracture dislocation in football. One or both malleoli may be fractured with dislocation of the talus and the obvious ligamentous rupture.

Stress Fracture This type of fracture occurs when the bone is under continual and prolonged stress – for example from the road running that is a part of many pre-season training programmes. The most common sites for stress fractures in football are the second metatarsal, the tibia and the fibula. There is rarely any incidence of significant trauma but rather a gradual and insidious onset of the following symptoms:

1. Pain during the latter stages of activity on hard surfaces.
2. Discoloration and localised swelling.
3. Pain experienced especially at night.
4. Discomfort when the site of injury is palpated.

TREATMENT OF FRACTURES

The first priority when treating a fracture on the field of play is immobilisation. Having established that your player has a fracture (the symptoms will probably include pain, deformity, effusion and complete lack of active movement) you must then start to immobilise the affected limb.

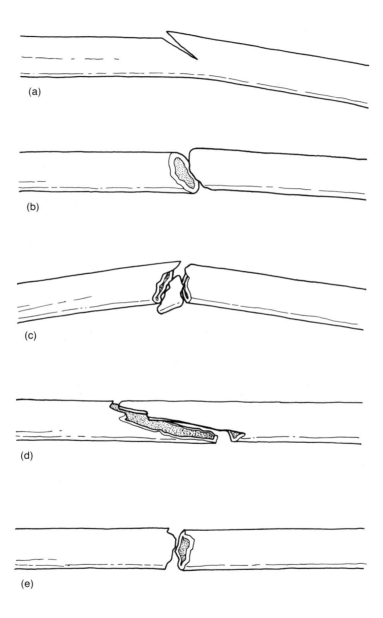

Fig 19 *Types of fracture; greenstick (a), transverse (b), angulated (c), spiral (d), oblique (e).*

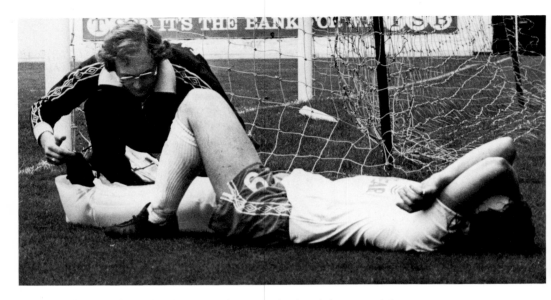

Fig 20 The use of an inflatable splint for an undisplaced fracture of the right fibula.

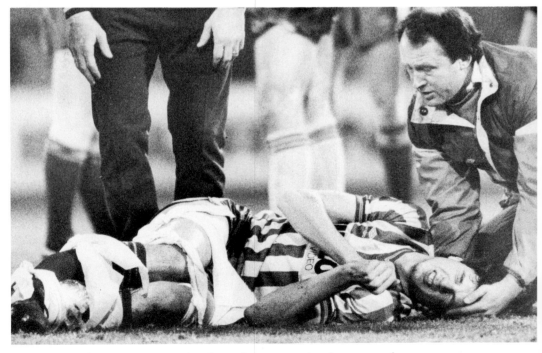

Fig 21 The use of triangular bandages for an angulated compound fracture of the right tibia and fibula.

If the player's fracture does not have any 'angulation', the best method to use is to apply an inflatable splint as shown in Fig 20 (this shows an undisplaced fracture of the fibula). In the case of an angulated fracture it is impractical to apply an inflatable splint and so the use of triangular bandages is required to immobilise the limb.

Place the sound leg next to the injured leg, and tie a figure of eight around both ankles and feet, starting the application with the bandage placed behind both Achilles tendons. Then fold the bandage across the front of both feet and tie on the sound side if possible using a reef-knot. The second bandage should be positioned below the site of the fracture, again secured on the sound leg by a reef-knot. A third and fourth bandage should be applied above the site of the fracture at distances suitable for giving support. (Fig 21 shows the immobilisation of an angulated fibula and tibia fracture.)

It is of the utmost importance that you ensure the materials necessary to immobilise a fracture are always available as well as a stretcher and whenever possible, an ambulance on call.

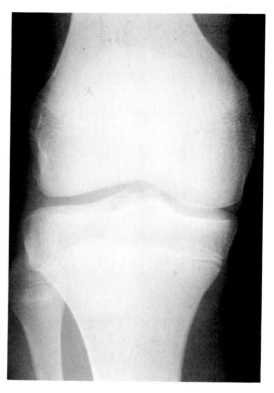

Fig 22 *An X-ray of the tibia of a fifteen-year-old footballer showing the epiphysis.*

INJURIES OF ADOLESCENCE

Separation of the Epiphysis

The epiphysis is the spongy extremity of a growing bone, is covered on its surface by cartilage and is developed from a distinct ossification (or process of bone growth). In the adolescent this spongy material is connected with the shaft of the bone by a plate of cartilage that gradually disappears as maturity is reached. Separation of the epiphysis from its bone is a form of fracture which sometimes occurs in the young footballer aged between ten and sixteen.

Other Conditions of Adolescence

Osgood–Schlatter's Disease

This condition arises when the epiphysis of the anterior tibial tubercle becomes damaged by the excessive pull from the ligamentum patellae (*see* Fig 23).

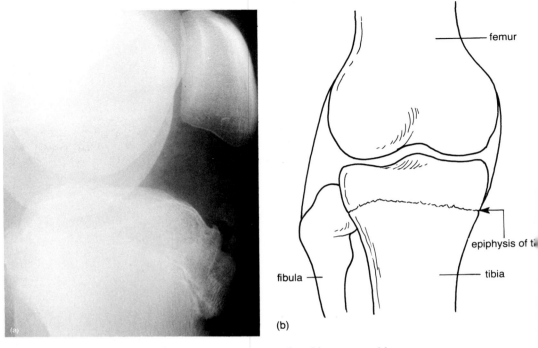

Fig 23   Osgood–Schlatter's disease: (a) an X-ray of a fifteen-year-old footballer and (b) a diagrammatic view of the knee joint showing the epiphysis of the tibia.

Sinding–Larsen–Johannson's Disease

This condition is rare compared with Osgood–Schlatter's disease and is an osteochondritis of the lower pole of the patella (*see* Fig 24).

Sever's Disease

The epiphysis of the calcaneum (heel bone) is affected by the pull of the Achilles' tendon (*see* Fig 25).

These conditions arise generally through overuse and not from direct contact. It is not uncommon for a young talented footballer to be subjected to greater participation than is good for him and so suffer from conditions

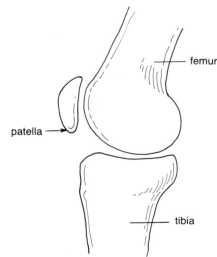

Fig 24   The diagram shows the area of the patella that is affected by the condition named Sinding–Larssen–Johansson's disease.

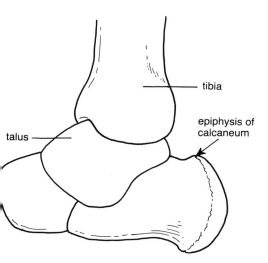

Fig 25   The diagram indicates the position of the epiphysis of the calcaneum. The condition related to this epiphyseal plate is named Sever's disease.

caused by overuse. If any young players report to you that they are experiencing pain during or after activity without having suffered direct contact, you should send them for a consultation with their doctor.

The treatment for these conditions in the severe stage is to immobilise the injured area in plaster. In cases which are not so far advanced, resting from activity is the best method to help the problem heal.

5 Muscular Injuries

ANATOMICAL CONSIDERATIONS

Each muscle has an origin and an insertion; the origin, under normal circumstances, remains fixed during the movement of the muscle, while the insertion, which is generally attached to bone, is the part that moves. Some muscles are directed obliquely and this anatomical positioning increases both the speed and power of their action. Muscles vary in shape depending on the arrangement of their fibres, for example the rectus femoris muscle of the quadriceps. This is known as a 'bipennate' muscle which means that its fibres arise from two tendinous heads. Each muscle has a good blood supply and also a nerve supply for both sensory and motor nerves.

Injuries to muscles either have an extrinsic cause (such as a direct blow) or an intrinsic cause (from overuse of a particular muscle or muscle group). An example of the latter is an intrinsic strain of the quadriceps muscle, the rectus femoris, which can occur during a prolonged shooting practice.

The muscles most commonly affected by intrinsic injury are those that affect the movement of two joints. The rectus femoris may serve again as an example as this muscle helps to perform both hip flexion and knee extension and so can be subject to intrinsic injury when kicking powerfully and sprinting vigor-

ously. The superficial muscles (nearest the surface) of the outer thigh and leg are prone to injury from extrinsic forces

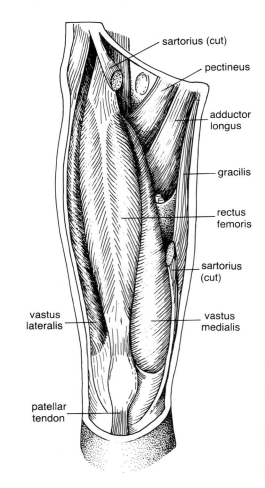

Fig 26 *The superficial muscles on the front of the thigh.*

34

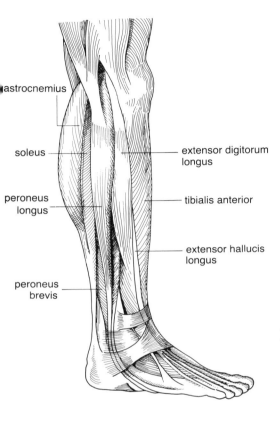

Fig 27 The superficial muscles on the lateral aspect of the leg.

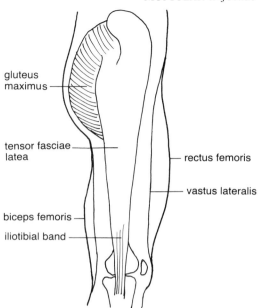

Fig 28 The muscles on the lateral aspect of the thigh.

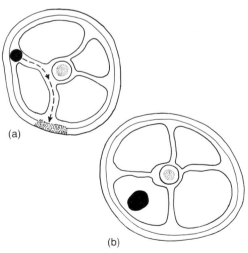

Fig 29 The intermuscular haematoma (a). The blood tracks down intermuscular fascial planes and appears as bruising some distance from the site of the original injury. The intramuscular haematoma (b) tends to absorb slowly and can usually be palpated.

The Haematoma

A muscle haematoma may be inter-muscular, intramuscular or combined. In the case of an intermuscular haematoma, blood passes down the inter-muscular fascial planes with the bruise often appearing some distance from the site of injury (*see* Fig 29a). With the intramuscular haematoma the swelling is more localised and the haematoma palpable; this type of muscle injury tends to absorb more slowly than the intermuscular (*see* Fig 29b).

35

DIAGNOSIS

As part of the diagnostic procedure you must ask the player how the injury occurred; 'Was it the result of a direct blow?', 'Do you think it was caused by overuse?' or 'Did you stretch awkwardly to control the ball?' The symptoms you will see will include pain, spasm, an inability either to contract the muscle or to stretch it without severe limitation and pain, tenderness to the touch and perhaps an obvious (palpable) swelling.

INTRINSIC MUSCLE INJURIES

There are three levels of intrinsic muscle injury: the first, the strain, involves only a few muscle fibres being stressed and the symptoms are relatively minor; the second – a serious injury – is the partial tear in which quite a number of muscle fibres are torn, producing more pronounced symptoms than the strain; the third level is the rupture when the muscle tears completely, leaving the player with gross limitations and extreme symptoms; a gap will be palpable in the muscle.

If a player ruptures his calf muscle (which would usually happen at the musculo-tendinous junction of gastrocnemius and soleus, see Fig 27) the player will feel as though he has been kicked in the calf or hit by an object – neither of which has actually happened. However, the muscle will have ruptured through a sudden intrinsic force and not from an extrinsic involvement.

Treatment

For the mild strain, normally reported at the end of the game, you should apply ice for a period of ten to fifteen minutes and then a modified pressure bandage consisting of two layers of hospital-quality cotton wool, each layer compressed by a 15cm (6in) crêpe bandage. Rest and elevation of the injured limb for a period of twenty-four hours should also be encouraged. If a player is suffering from a partial tear he will have had to leave the field, will be in considerable pain and will have an obvious limitation of function. The same procedure should be followed for the immediate treatment of this degree of injury – ice, pressure, rest and elevation of the injured limb. The rest period should be extended to forty-eight hours.

For a ruptured muscle the symptoms are extreme; the player will have no active movement and will be in excruciating pain. He must be taken from the field on a stretcher and immediately transported to hospital. Surgery is normally required for this level of injury.

EXTRINSIC MUSCLE INJURIES

There are two levels of extrinsic muscle injury: the first, a contusion or bruise, is quite superficial and absorbs ('goes down') quickly; the second is a haematoma, which may be of the intermuscular or intramuscular type. When there is a haematoma, muscle tissue, blood vessels, sensory and motor nerves are all involved, meaning that the trauma (and the resulting pain) can be quite severe and the ability to stretch the muscle is limited according to the severity of injury.

Treatment

For a contusion you should first apply an ice-pack for the usual ten to fifteen minutes and use a tubigrip support over the affected area. A twenty-four hour period of rest and elevation should then be sufficient for this type of injury to settle down.

In the case of haematoma, an ice-pack as well as a complete pressure bandage and forty-eight hours of rest and elevation of the injured limb will be required. To aid recovery, the club doctor or the player's general practitioner may perhaps prescribe a course of anti-inflammatory tablets accompanied by physiotherapy and gradual rehabilitation.

6 Knee Injuries

The Anatomy of the Knee Joint

The knee joint comprises the lower end of the femur, the upper part of the tibia and the patella. The ends of these bones are known as condyles and so the articulation (or movement) of the knee joint is between the condyles of the femur and the condyles of the tibia and also between the lower end of the femur and the patella (*see* Fig 31).

The knee joint is of the synovial type because of its numerous synovial bursae (sacs which contain synovial fluid, a lubricant). The joint between the femur and the tibia is an atypical hinge joint because it allows a degree of rotation and the joint between the femur and patella is an atypical plane joint since gliding is not the only movement that takes place there. There are a number of structures that ought to be fully considered so far as their anatomy is concerned because the injury risk to these areas is quite high in football.

Ligamentum Patellae

The ligamentum patellae extends from the apex of the patella and downwards on to the tibial tubercle. It is separated from the synovial membrane by the infrapatellar pad of fat and from the upper part of the tibia by the infrapatellar bursa (*see* Fig 31).

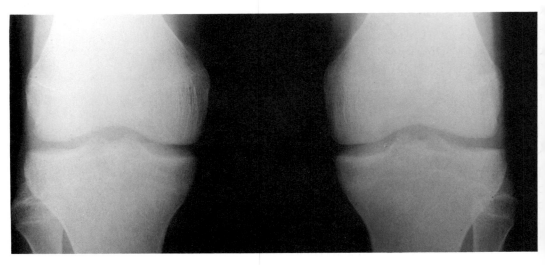

Fig 30   An X-ray of the knee joints.

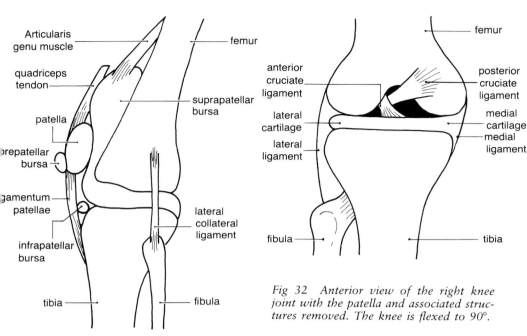

Fig 32 *Anterior view of the right knee joint with the patella and associated structures removed. The knee is flexed to 90°.*

Fig 31 *Bursae in relation to the knee joint; a side (lateral) view.*

The Lateral Collateral Ligament

This ligament is attached to the lateral condyle of the femur, passes downwards over the joint line on to the head of the fibula. It is a very strong cord-like structure.

The Medial Collateral Ligament

The upper attachment is to the medial condyle of the femur. This structure is broad and flat, its deeper fibres at joint-line level attach to the medial cartilage. The ligament passes downwards from the joint line on to the medial tibial condyle (*see* Fig 32).

The Cruciate Ligaments

The two cruciate ligaments are termed anterior (front) and posterior (back) according to their tibial attachments and they are very strong – the rupture of one or both of these ligaments results in an unstable knee joint (*see* Fig 32).

The Anterior Cruciate Ligament

The anterior cruciate ligament is attached to the anterior intercondyloid area of the tibia and passes upwards and backwards to be attached to the posterior part of the medial surface of the lateral condyle of the femur. The anterior cruciate ligament prevents over-extension of the knee joint.

39

The Posterior Cruciate Ligament

The posterior cruciate ligament is attached to the posterior intercondyloid area of the tibia and passes upwards and forwards to be attached to the anterior part of the lateral surface of the medial condyle of the femur. The posterior cruciate ligament keeps the tibia in contact with the femur in flexion (*see* Fig 32).

The Semilunar Cartilages or Menisci

There are two of these cartilages in each knee joint, the medial (inside) cartilage and the lateral (outside) cartilage. Their shape is semilunar or semicircular with the surface in contact with the tibia flat and the surface in contact with the femur concave. A side view of the cartilage is roughly triangular, and when viewed from above the shape is semilunar.

The menisci are attached to the tibia at its periphery by the coronary ligaments and also by a band of fibrous tissue called the transverse ligament. Menisci effectively act as the shock absorbers in the knee joint, contribute to the joint's stability and help to absorb synovial fluid.

The Lateral Cartilage or Meniscus

The lateral cartilage is attached by its anterior horn to the anterior intercondylar area on the tibia immediately in front of the intercondylar eminence, and

by its posterior horn to the posterior intercondylar area. Some fibres of the popliteus muscle are attached to the posterior area of the lateral meniscus either directly or through the arcuate ligament, so giving a small degree of mobility.

The Medial Cartilage or Meniscus

The positioning of this cartilage is broadly similar to the lateral meniscus. The major anatomical difference is that the medial meniscus is less mobile than its lateral counterpart because deeper fibres of the medial ligament are attached to the meniscus (*see* Fig 33).

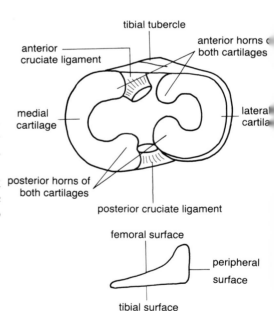

Fig 33 A superior view of the tibial condyles to show the position and surface shape of the cartilages (menisci).

The Articularis Genu Muscle

The articularis genu muscle tenses the suprapatellar bursa when the knee is extended and prevents the synovial membrane being nipped between the femur and the patella.

INJURIES TO THE KNEE JOINT

The Torn Cartilage

The most common cause of a torn cartilage is a weight-bearing rotational force, for example when the femur presses downwards on to the fixed tibia and tears the cartilage. This can produce the most frequently experienced cartilage injury, the 'bucket-handle' tear in which a central segment of cartilage or meniscus is displaced and floats into the centre of the joint – greatly increasing the possibility that the knee could 'lock'.

If you are presented with the most common type of cartilage injury, you will probably see the following symptoms: the player will be unable to straighten his knee; the joint will feel unstable; the active range of flexion and extension would be severely limited. The correct procedure is to remove the player from the field of play on a stretcher with his knee (or knees) immobilised. If the knee is not fully extended use triangular bandages to fix the legs together, tying a figure of eight around the ankles and two single bandages just below and just above the knee. Do not attempt to move the fixed position of the joint as this would remove valuable clinical 'evidence'.

Having removed the player from the field discuss with him exactly how his injury occurred. As a guideline the following question and answer procedure will be of value to you in helping you to make an accurate diagnosis.

1. 'Was there a click, snap or tearing sensation within the joint?'
2. Location of pain. 'Is the pain medial (on the inside) of the knee or lateral (on the outer side) of the joint?'
3. 'Do you experience locking of the joint?' If so, 'in what position was the joint when this happened?'
4. Swelling or effusion. 'Was the swelling immediate or not?'
5. Check for any temperature in the joint by feeling the knee joint in both hands and comparing with the sound knee.
6. 'Does the knee feel as if it will give way and in what circumstances?'
7. 'Can you extend the knee actively?'
8. 'Can you flex the knee actively?'
9. McMurray's manoeuvre should only be performed by a physiotherapist, doctor or specialist once having transported the player to hospital.

Causes of Injury to the Ligaments

The most common mechanics of injury to the medial collateral ligament is the 'valgus', caused by stress or by direct contact in which the joint is forced into the 'knock-kneed' position. The lateral collateral ligament can be injured by a 'varus' or 'bow-leg' stress or direct contact. If the anterior cruciate ligament alone is injured, the knee joint is forced into hyperextension. If only the posterior cruciate ligament is injured, the knee is forced into flexion.

The Degrees of Injury
The Mild Sprain

The usual symptoms are as follows: a full range of active knee flexion and extension, a mild level of discomfort, no swelling and no redness or temperature in the joint – the player is able to continue in the game after a cold application.

The Moderate Sprain

The pain is increased, active movement is restricted and a swelling may be detectable. A player showing these symptoms should be removed from the field of play and professional medical advice sought.

The Rupture

The player will be in excruciating pain, there will be no active movement present and a haemarthrosis (blood entering the joint) will be detectable by feeling both knees for a difference in temperature caused by the blood from the ruptured ligament tissue entering the knee joint. This injury should be treated as though it were a fracture and the player must be taken to hospital immediately.

CLINICAL EXAMINATION OF THE KNEE JOINT

When examining an injured knee joint it is very important to compare it with the sound joint. In so doing, you can establish the normal ligament length and joint stability and discover the degree of injury. It is also essential to find out from the player whether or not there has been a history of injuries to the knee.

One method of examination is to feel (or 'palpate') the injured structure – if this is anatomically possible. Another method is for you to subject the structure of the knee to gentle stress by performing movements that increase the length of the ligament. These tests must be carried out with the muscle groups relaxed and you must also ensure that the movement is neither hurried nor vigorous. If the player experiences pain or if you feel an abnormal movement (in comparison to the sound knee) this indicates injury to a particular ligament. To palpate the injury is preferable since this should, to a large degree, isolate the site of the injury. Because it is quite common for more than one ligament to be damaged in an injury, a comprehensive comparative examination should always be carried out.

The Medial Collateral Ligament

In the dressing-room, the player lies on his back on the treatment plinth while the trainer stands on the lateral (outside) of the knee. One hand is placed on the inner side of the leg just above the ankle and the other just above the knee on the outside of the base of the thigh. The leg is lifted with the knee flexed at 15°–20°. Gentle pressure is applied to draw the leg outwards while the knee is pressed inwards into the valgus (or knock-kneed) position.

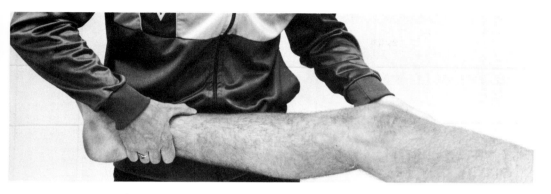

Fig 34 The stress test for the medial collateral ligament of the knee joint.

The Lateral Collateral Ligament

The player lies on the treatment plinth with the trainer standing by the outer side of the knee joint. One hand is positioned on the inside of the knee above the joint and the other on the outside of the lower leg just above the ankle. The knee is pressed outwards into the varus (or bow-legged) position. Once again this test is performed with the knee in a flexed position of 15°–20° as by doing this the stability of the joint is wholly dependent upon whichever collateral ligament you choose to test. A valgus or varus stress-test performed with the knee in full extension would not be accurate since under these circumstances both cruciate ligaments exert a stabilising influence.

The Cruciate Ligaments

The player lies on the treatment plinth on his back with the knee joint flexed at about 90°. The foot is positioned flat on the couch so that the trainer can sit on

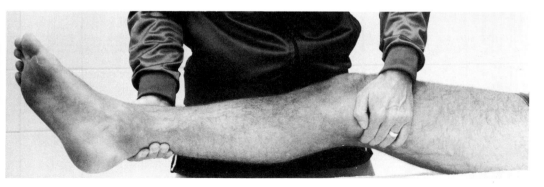

Fig 35 The stress test for the lateral collateral ligament of the knee joint.

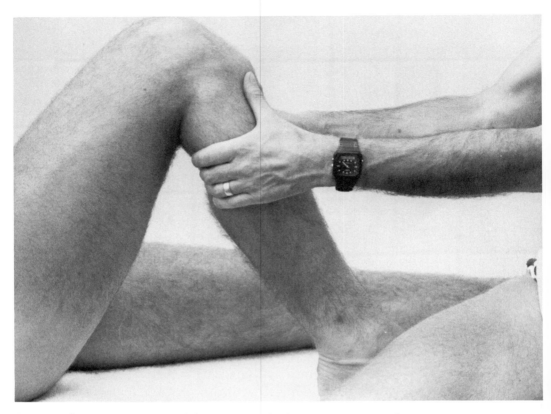

Fig 36 *The starting position of the stress test for both the anterior and posterior cruciate ligaments.*

it to anchor the tibia before examination. The tibia is held in both hands just below the condyles with the thumbs situated either side of the tibial tubercle.

The Anterior and Posterior Cruciate Ligaments

To test the anterior ligament, the tibia is drawn towards the trainer in a forward movement (the anterior draw sign) and in order to test the posterior ligament, the tibia is pushed backwards to produce the posterior draw sign. It is of vital importance when testing the ligaments that all the muscles are completely relaxed.

TYPES OF INFLAMMATION AND SWELLING

Effusions of the knee joint An effusion is the general term used to describe the condition in which there is excessive fluid in a joint. There are a number of different types of effusion.

Synovitis This is inflammation of the synovial membrane following a direct blow or injury to the menisci. It is a slow swelling that usually appears over a period of twelve to twenty-four hours. The most prominent effusion is situated around the suprapatellar bursa.

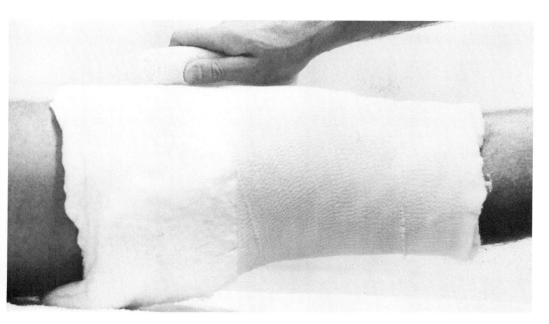

Fig 37   The application of a pressure bandage for the knee joint: the first crêpe bandage is wound over the first layer of cotton wool.

Haemarthrosis Increased temperature is a symptom of a haemarthrosis because of the blood content in the fluid of the joint. This type of effusion is immediate and may result from a fracture within the joint, ligament rupture or a direct blow that has ruptured blood vessels.

Bursitis Bursitis (the swelling of a bursa) is a localised inflammation brought about by a direct blow or repeated irritation. Because the function of bursae is to act as cushions between tendon and bone, they are especially vulnerable to injury. The most commonly injured bursa in the knee is the pre-patellar bursa.

The Compression

After consultation and examination you will have concluded exactly what is injured and the severity of this injury. In the case of a first or second-degree ligament injury or a torn cartilage that has not locked, a full compression bandage should be used after you have administered ice:

First apply a full turn around the knee of hospital-quality cotton wool, so that it covers three finger widths above the apex of the patella and no lower than the tibial tubercle. Then using a crêpe bandage of width 15cm (6in), apply two turns at joint level and two turns below the knee, leaving exposed a piece of cotton wool of 2cm (¾in) in width. Continue your turns of crêpe bandage upwards, always covering half of the previous layer of crêpe until you again have 2cm of cotton wool showing at the top. Repeat this procedure twice more until you have a pressure bandage consisting of three layers of cotton wool, each layer compressed by crêpe

45

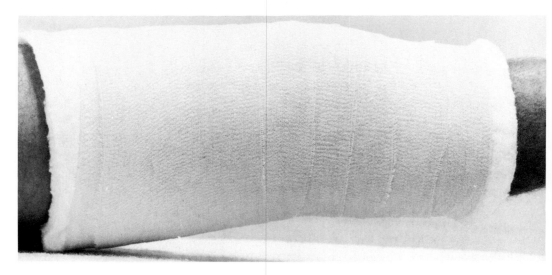

Fig 38 The completed pressure bandage for the knee joint.

bandage, finally tied down with elasto-plast strapping of width 7.5cm (3in).

The compression bandage is kept in position for a period of 24–48 hours depending on the severity of the injury. When applying the crêpe, increase the pressure of application gradually, with little pressure on the first turns over the first piece of cotton wool, more pressure in applying the second and then firm pressure on the third and final stage. Check the circulation is adequate by pressing your finger against the tibia and note how quickly the colour returns; then compare with the sound leg.

7 Ankle Injuries

ANATOMICAL CONSIDERATIONS

In order to be able to treat correctly any injury of the ankle joint, an accurate diagnosis must be made. This in turn requires a working knowledge of the anatomy of the ankle region. Let us consider those anatomical characteristics of the ankle that are directly relevant to the types of injury likely to occur in soccer as a result of the various forces to which it is subjected.

The ankle joint is functionally a hinge joint with movement in one plane. Flexion may either be plantar (toes pointed forwards) or dorsi (toes pointed upwards). The structure of the joint is of a similar design to a mortise and tenon and so has considerable stability. The 'mortise' is formed by the inner surface of the medial malleolus, the distal (lower) end of the tibia and the inner surface of the lateral malleolus (*see* Fig 40). The 'tenon' is formed by the body of the talus which is shaped to fit into the mortise.

The Lateral and Medial Malleoli

The lateral malleolus is longer than the medial malleolus and its distal tip ends at the bottom of the talus at the level of the talocalcaneal joint. Roughly rectangular in shape, it is, however, slightly

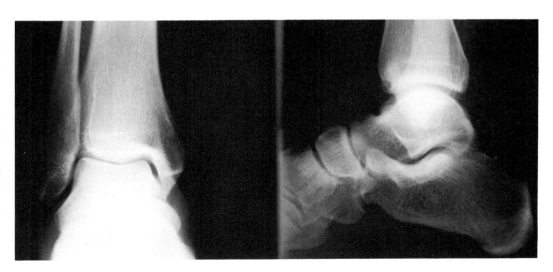

Fig 39   An X-ray of the ankle joint.

47

narrower at its lower end. The medial malleolus, on the other hand, is short and thick, being roughly pyramidal in shape with its base upwards. Its distal tip extends only half-way down the body of the talus.

Ligaments

The distal ends of the tibia and fibula are bound together by the anterior (front) and posterior (back) tibiofibular ligaments which are thickened expansions of the interosseous membrane. The ankle joint has stability from two major sources; the 'mortise and tenon' structure of the bones and the large number of ligaments that surround the joint.

The ligaments are relatively thin in the anterior (front) and posterior (back) areas of the joint but they become thicker and stronger as the tibial and fibular deltoid ligaments develop on the medial (inside) and lateral (outside) aspects of the ankle. The medial deltoid ligament is very strong, has a very broad attachment to the medial or internal malleolus and extends downwards in three major ligamentous bands. In addition to stabilising the ankle joint on the medial side, it serves to support the arch of the foot. The medial deltoid ligament is triangular in shape and is attached by its apex to the medial malleolus. It then splits into three bands, the front attached to the tuberosity (prominent area) of the navicular bone, the middle to the spring ligament, the sustentaculum tali and finally the back to the talus (*see* Fig 41). The lateral deltoid ligament is attached to the medial aspect of the lateral malleolus and it too divides into three bands, the front passing forwards to the talus (called the anterior talofibular ligament) the middle passing downwards to the calcaneum (the calcaneofibular ligament) and the posterior, which is attached to the talus. The lateral deltoid ligament is

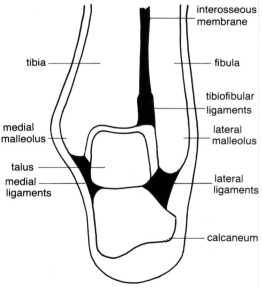

Fig 40   A diagrammatic anterior/posterior view of the ankle showing the bone structure of the joint and the major ligamentous attachments.

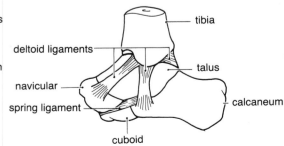

Fig 41   The ankle joint, medial aspect.

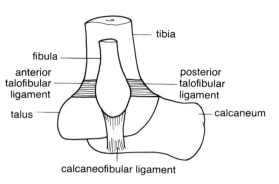

Fig 42   *The ankle joint, lateral aspect.*

clinically important because a damaged anterior talofibular ligament is the most common ankle injury in football (*see* Fig 42).

CAUSES OF INJURY

The Inversion Injury

Injuries usually result from the ankle joint being forced into plantar flexion (toes pointing forwards) and also into inversion, which means that the foot is forced inwards. It will be noted that the push is against the medial malleolus and the pull is away from the lateral malleolus. This mechanism puts a strain on the lateral ligament, the primary purpose of which is to restrict this movement. As a result of this over-inversion the ligament will tear slightly, partially or completely – according to the severity of force applied.

Approximately eighty-five per cent of all mild or first-degree sprains are inversion injuries and are confined to ligament injury. The moderate injury is, of course, a little more severe, but again will be a pure ligament injury. In the

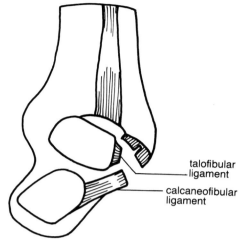

Fig 43   *A diagrammatic view of an inversion mechanism of the ankle joint producing a rupture of the lateral ligaments.*

case of complete rupture of the ligament there may well be associated fractures of either of the malleoli or even of the talus.

The Eversion Injury

To a certain extent the opposite mechanism applies here in that the ankle can be in dorsiflexion, toes pointing upwards (or more commonly in plantar flexion, toes pointing downwards) when the foot is forced outwards in eversion towards the lateral side. The talus is driven forcibly against the lateral malleolus and severe pressure is applied to the malleolus before stressing the medial deltoid ligaments. The severity of injury, of course, depends upon the force applied and once again the ligaments can be injured to three differing degrees, mild (sprain), moderate (partial tear) or severe (rupture).

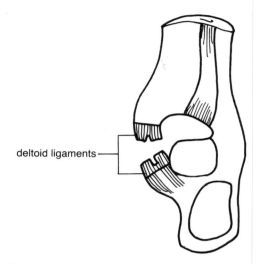

Fig 44   A diagrammatic view of an eversion injury of the ankle joint showing a rupture of the medial ligament.

deltoid ligaments

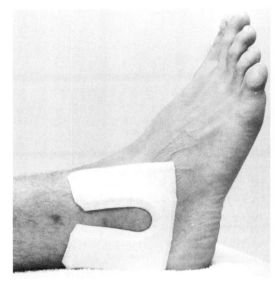

Fig 45   The pressure pad for a first-degree sprain of the lateral ligament of the ankle joint.

TREATMENT FOR INJURIES

Before treatment can be properly begun in any particular case, it is important to classify the injury not only according to the type and structures damaged but also to the severity.

The Mild Injury

The first degree of injury is the mild sprain which is normally reported after the game has finished – only occasionally is first aid required on the field. In this situation a ligament will have been stretched slightly beyond its normal range. There will be very little swelling and only mild pain in the extreme position of plantar flexion and of inversion (the most common mechanism of injury to the ankle joint).

The first treatment is to apply ice for

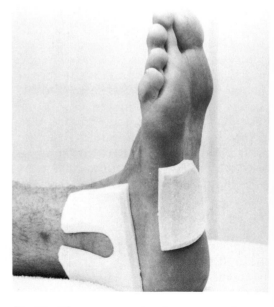

Fig 46   The support pad and pressure pad in position.

a period of ten to fifteen minutes, making sure the skin is protected from possible burns by smearing olive oil over the injured area before applying the ice-pack. At this stage heat of any kind should be avoided and the player encouraged to shower rather than bathe in hot water as this would open already damaged blood vessels so causing greater swelling. While the player is taking a quick shower the ice-pack and compression bandage can be prepared. Once the ice has been removed the ankle is compressed by a pad shaped to the contours of the joint as shown in Fig 45. A pad is then applied underneath

the foot (*see* Fig 46) in alignment with the lateral ligament to avoid further pressure which might accidently aggravate the injury. A comfortable but firm figure-of-eight strapping of either crêpe bandage or of elastoplast (7.5cm or 3in wide) is then applied for support.

Start the bandaging at the part of the foot closest to the toes and make two turns to anchor the bandage at this level. Next pull the bandage up and around the back of the ankle, applying a little extra pressure to keep the ankle in a position of dorsiflexion and the foot in eversion (*see* Fig 47). By positioning the ankle and foot in this

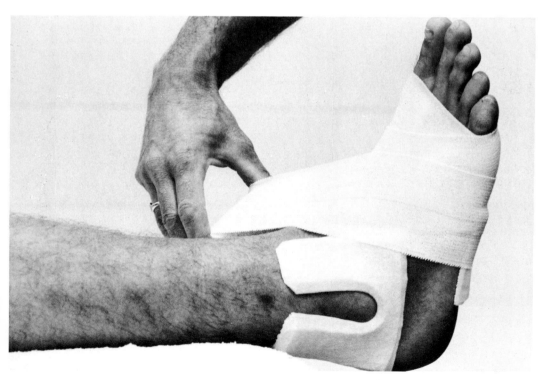

Fig 47 The application of the elastoplast strapping. Note the position of the first turns of the bandage and the start of the figure-of-eight application.

51

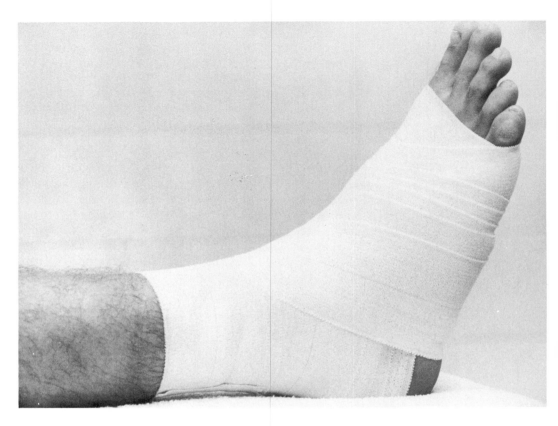

Fig 48   The completed pressure bandage for a first-degree sprain of the lateral ligament of the ankle joint.

manner the ligament is encouraged to heal quickly and efficiently. Continue winding the bandage around the ankle in a figure of eight and finish the compression with two neat turns above the ankle joint (Fig 48). The player should be told to rest and elevate the ankle for a period of twenty-four hours.

The Moderate Injury

The second degree of injury is the moderate or partial tear. The player will not be able to continue in the game having sustained this degree of injury. A noticeable swelling will be evident, as well as a limited active range of move-

ment and a considerable amount of pain. Following the application of ice the player should not take any weight on the injured ankle so ensure he has a pair of crutches so that he can carry out your instructions to the full. As a rule moderate ankle ligament injuries should always be X-rayed in case there is a fracture. Once this possibility has been eliminated, the injured ankle should be rested and elevated for a period of forty-eight hours with the ankle compressed by a full-pressure bandage consisting of three layers of hospital-quality cotton wool, each layer compressed by a crêpe bandage and finally tied down with elastoplast strapping.

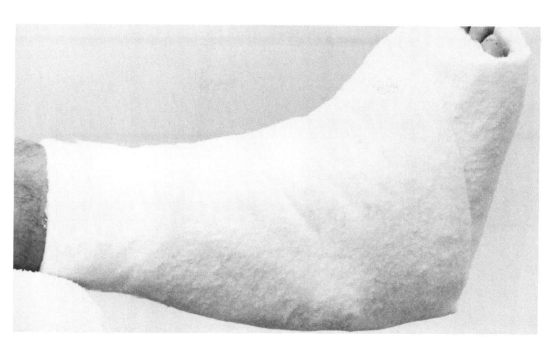

Fig 49   The first layer of hospital-quality cotton wool is applied.

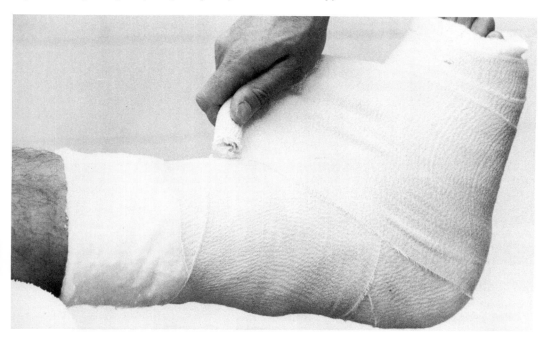

Fig 50   Next, apply the first covering of crêpe bandage. Again, note the position of the turns and the figure-of-eight manoeuvre.

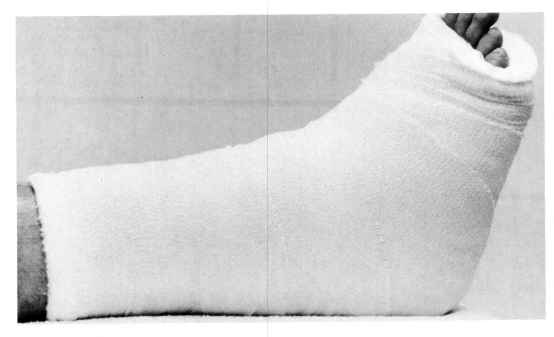

Fig 51   The completed pressure bandage for a second-degree sprain of the lateral ligament of the ankle joint.

The Severe Injury

The third degree of ankle injury usually involves a rupture of a ligament. This, the most serious of ligament injuries to the ankle joint, could well be accompanied by a fracture or dislocation. If you meet this injury it will be on the field of play, and the player will be suffering excruciating pain. There will be no active movement, and immediate swelling and an increase in temperature in the joint caused by haemarthrosis. The player may believe that he has a fracture. The important point with an injury of this severity is to immobilise the ankle. This can be achieved either by using an inflatable splint (Fig 20) or by the use of triangular bandages. If you are using the latter, the technique is to tie a figure of eight around both the ankles with a cushion between the feet,

then tie a second bandage roughly in line with the middle of the calves and finally a third just above the knees. Having completed the immobilisation, remove the player from the field on a stretcher and transport him to hospital.

It is very important to remember that you must *not* give a drink to any player who requires hospital treatment since he may need an anaesthetic. This will not be immediately possible if the patient has recently consumed any food or drink.

THE ACHILLES TENDON

The Achilles tendon is located at the back of the ankle and is a thick, cord-like structure of great strength. It is a continuation of the gastrocnemius

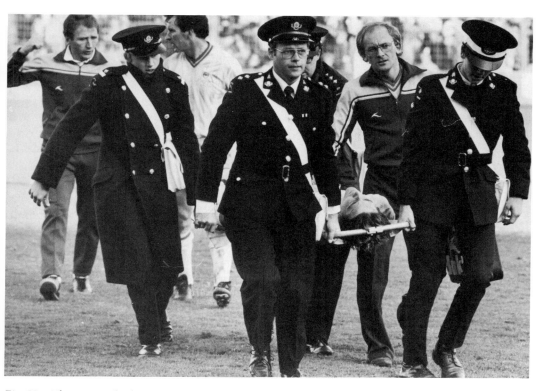

Fig 52   The removal of a player from the field on a stretcher. Note the ambulance men in comfortable carrying positions, with the physiotherapist in close attendance, supervising the operation.

muscle (the major muscle in the calf) and of the soleus (beneath the gastrocnemius).

In soccer the Achilles tendon is injured either by a direct kick, producing a contusion or haematoma, depending on the severity of the blow, or by overuse. In both cases you should follow the principles of initial treatment: application of ice; compression; rest; and elevation. An excellent – and simple – form of treatment for injury to the Achilles tendon is to place a felt pad into the heel of the player's shoe. This will elevate and slightly shorten the tendon, so relieving stress and strain when walking.

The most common 'mechanisms' for injury are for the player to be sprinting (or starting to sprint) or perhaps jumping to head the ball – in each case he pushes down with the toes of one foot, so putting considerable pressure on the tendon. If he has partially torn or ruptured his Achilles tendon, the symptoms are acute and immediate.

Symptoms and Treatment

So far as symptoms are concerned, the player who has partially ruptured his Achilles tendon will be in great pain. He will feel as though he has been violently kicked (or hit by a heavy object) in the calf – whereas in reality he has felt the tissue of the Achilles tendon rupturing.

The range of plantar flexion of the ankle joint will be severely limited and although the range of dorsiflexion will not be much reduced, movement will be exceptionally painful. Additionally, the tendon will be very tender on palpation and any resistance to the movement of plantar flexion will be excruciating.

A player who has completely ruptured his Achilles tendon will display extreme symptoms; he will be in agony and while unable to manage any range of plantar flexion, the range of dorsiflexion will be greater than normal. Moreover, there will be a visible gap in the tendon at the site of rupture. A test for the integrity of the tendon is to squeeze the gastrocnemius muscle and compare the extent of the plantar flexion with the sound ankle when gripped in the same manner; if there is a rupture, the range of movement of the injured ankle will be grossly curtailed.

The first-aid treatment for the casualty who has either partially or completely ruptured his Achilles tendon is to remove the player from the field and to take him by ambulance to hospital. This is a serious injury and must be given immediate professional medical attention.

8 Foot Injuries

ANATOMICAL CONSIDERATIONS

The bones of the foot comprise the tarsal, metatarsal and phalangeal bones. The tarsal bones are made up of the calcaneum, talus, navicular, cuboid and three cuneiform bones (*see* Fig 53). The calcaneum articulates above with the talus and to the front with the cuboid. The medial surface presents a prominence of bone named the sustentaculum tali. The talus articulates with both the tibia and fibula above, with the calcaneum below and with the navicular bone to the front.

The remaining tarsal bones are the cuboid, the navicular and the three cuneiform (wedge-shaped) bones which are situated immediately in front of the navicular bone. These are termed medial (inside) intermediate (middle) and lateral (outside), according to their anatomical position. The metatarsals and phalanges are arranged in a manner similar to the bones of the hand. The bones are firmly bound together by ligaments running from the front of the talus to the metatarsal heads. The general contour of the foot is a longitudinal arch resting at the back on the bottom of the calcaneum and at the front on the metatarsal heads. This arch is supported by the very strong plantar ligament which extends from the calcaneum forwards to attach itself close to the metatarsal heads. The bones of

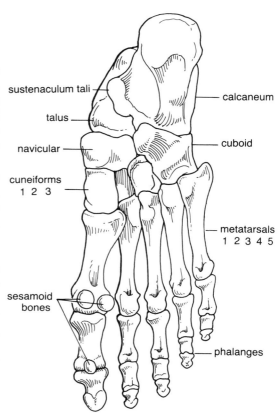

Fig 53 The bones of the right foot viewed from below.

the foot have many ligamentous and tendinous attachments, creating a rather complex anatomy.

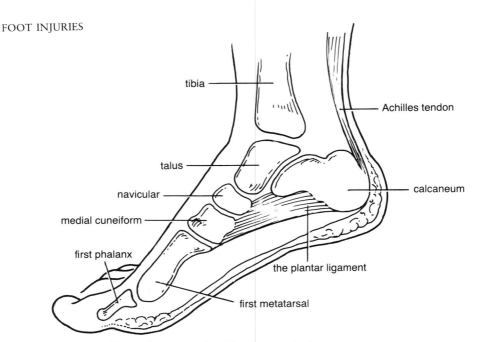

Fig 54   A section of the right foot and ankle showing the bony structure. The Achilles tendon and plantar ligament can also be seen.

INJURIES

Contusions

A contusion to the foot is a frequent occurrence in soccer and may often be caused by a direct blow; a player's foot may be stamped on or perhaps kicked. The symptoms, normally reported after the game, will essentially be nothing more than that the foot is painful to walk on. In your examination you will detect localised swelling, discoloration of the affected area and finally an unimpeded active range of movement. The pain will be localised to the site where direct contact was made.

The basic principles of treatment should be put into operation once you have diagnosed a contusion. Apply an ice-pack after placing a protective covering for the foot between the skin and the ice. While the ice is in position, cut a piece of surgical felt to the shape and size of the affected area. You should also cut some elastoplast strapping of width 7.5cm (3in) or a crêpe bandage of the same size. Remove the ice-pack after the recommended period of time has elapsed and place the surgical felt in position on the foot. If there is a wound, this must, of course, be thoroughly cleaned and a sterile dressing applied before the surgical felt.

The bandage application may either be around the foot or in a figure-of-eight technique, depending upon the site of the contusion. Tell the player to rest and elevate his foot for a period of twenty-four hours.

Sprains

The ligaments of the foot are sprained by being stretched beyond their normal stabilising range. The most common cause is a forced plantar flexion (toes straight out) of the ankle joint which stretches the ligaments and tendons on the top of the foot. The incident in soccer that most often produces this type of injury is when a player attempts to strike the ball and finds it completely blocked by an opponent. It may also occur when a player accidentally kicks the ground rather than the ball. This injury will, of course, be mild, moderate or severe and the symptoms include pain, a reduced active range of movement and immediate swelling (in the case of a moderate or severe injury). If a player has suffered a mild sprain, he will usually report the injury after the game has finished.

In the case of a moderate injury you will be required to diagnose the player's injury on the pitch but he will be unable to continue the game because of pain and limitation of function. Having removed him from the field of play, apply the basic principles of first-aid treatment as usual; ice, compression, rest and elevation of the injured limb until physiotherapy can be organised for the injured player.

The third and most serious degree of injury – the rupture – will have the same symptoms as a fracture; the player will be in extreme pain and an immediate swelling will be present, accompanied by a gross loss of active movement. He may well believe that he has suffered a fracture. The treatment on the field of play is for the trainer to immobilise the foot as for a fracture, transport the player to hospital by ambulance for X-ray examination and specialist treatment.

Fractures

In soccer the bones of the foot are fractured by two distinct mechanisms; direct contact and overuse (producing stress fractures).

In the past one of my players has fractured the navicular through direct contact; metatarsals also may be fractured by a severe direct blow. The fifth metatarsal is most commonly fractured in this manner while the second, third and fourth are more likely to suffer from a stress fracture.

If the fifth metatarsal has been fractured as a result of a direct kick the symptoms will include pain, limited active foot movement, swelling and tenderness to the touch. Most such fractures are undisplaced but if the symptoms are as previously mentioned, the player must be taken to hospital for an X-ray examination.

A stress fracture is most likely to occur in the metatarsal region. The onset of pain is gradual and will be particularly uncomfortable after activity on hard surfaces. An X-ray may not initially show the site of the fracture, although it will become evident after a number of weeks, when the X-ray will show the callus development gradually appearing.

Strains

A strain of the plantar ligament is not uncommon in soccer. If a player complains of pain in the arch of his foot when running and has not been kicked there, it is advisable to substitute the player concerned for examination and initial treatment. His doctor may well recommend a course of physiotherapy.

Tenosynovitis

The foot is often prone to tenosynovitis because its tendons are responsible not only for movement but also for supporting considerable body weight. The cause is the same as in other areas of the body, namely a direct blow or chronic overuse. Frequently tenosynovitis is combined with a tendon strain or a haematoma. The resulting irritation causes friction between the tendon and its surrounding sheath producing inflammation and adhesions, all of which cause pain during active function of the foot. Careful palpation over the tendon while active movement is carried out will often detect crepitus or creaking, which is symptomatic of tenosynovitis.

The treatment in the initial stage is to apply ice, compress, rest and elevate the injured foot. An appointment should be made with the club or the player's doctor and a request for physiotherapy made to him or her if he feels the need to do so. Exercise should not be resumed until the symptoms have fully cleared.

Fractures of the Toes

The first or 'big' toe should be considered separately since it is much more important in the mechanics of the foot than the other, smaller toes. The toe may be injured by a direct blow, causing a very painful injury with considerable bleeding into the tissues, swelling, throbbing and severe discomfort. If a fracture is suspected, an X-ray examination is required at hospital to determine whether there is a fracture involving the joint since this has much more serious implications than a fracture of the shaft alone. Indeed, if you are presented with any toe injury which has similar symptoms to those mentioned above, do not hesitate to take the player to hospital for an X-ray.

Conditions of the Foot

The Verruca

The verruca or wart is a viral skin disease and can spread over the foot, becoming very disabling if not diagnosed, treated and eradicated early. Treatment, in hospital, should only be carried out by people especially proficient in the treatment of such conditions.

Corns

The best way to avoid any form of disability in a footballer from a corn is to prevent the corn occurring at all. Shoes and boots must always fit correctly and even wrinkles in a sock can contribute to the onset of a corn. The most common site for a corn is on the outer surface of the little toe; an appointment with the local chiropodist is advisable if a player has developed a corn.

Athlete's Foot

Fungal infections of the foot are not uncommon in the dressing-room and shower area of a soccer club. The surface of the skin between the toes peels, leaving a red, sore area. Encourage your players to wear flip-flops in the shower and dressing-room areas and persuade them to dry thoroughly between the toes before applying a powder such as Mycil or Tinaderm.

Ingrown Toe-Nails

An ingrown toe-nail may occur in any toe but is most common and severe in the first toe. Put simply, the cause is a rolling of the toe nail in a scroll-like fashion so that the two outer edges tend to roll closer to the toe than the rest of the nail, forming a semi-circular tube rather than a flat plane. The resulting convexity causes the edge of the nail to dig into the side of the toe, making the toe very sore and painful. The treatment for this condition should be carried out by a chiropodist (although *see* Chapter 1 for prevention).

Bruised Toe-Nail

A bruised toe-nail is commonly received in soccer either from a direct blow or gradually from the first toe and nail repeatedly being compressed against the end of the player's boot. The pain can be quite considerable and the treatment, which should be carried out only by a medically qualified person, is gradually to pierce the nail with a sterile needle. Having reached the haematoma, the release of blood produces a great relief from pain.

9 Shoulder Injuries

ANATOMICAL CONSIDERATIONS

The shoulder joint is a synovial ball-and-socket joint. The joint's articulation is between the head of the humerus and the shallow glenoid cavity of the scapula (shoulder-blade). The glenoid cavity is deepened by the labrum which is attached to its margins and is an intracapsular structure. The capsule of the shoulder is reinforced at the front (anterior) by the three glenohumeral ligaments called, according to their anatomical position, superior, middle and inferior (*see* Fig 57). These ligaments provide stability for the shoulder and prevent excessive movement. The coracohumeral ligament strengthens the capsule from above and attaches to the coracoid process of the scapula and to the greater tuberosity of the humerus (*see* Fig 57). The muscles that form the rotator cuff also strengthen the capsule. The synovial membrane lines the capsule to cover the glenoid labrum and the long head of the muscle biceps.

The Sternoclavicular Joint

The articulation of the sternoclavicular joint is between the clavicle (collarbone), the upper part of the sternum and the first costal cartilage. The joint is

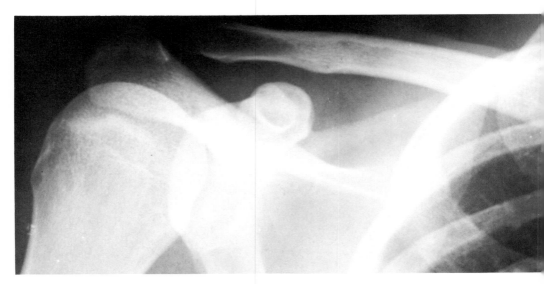

Fig 55   An X-ray of the shoulder joint.

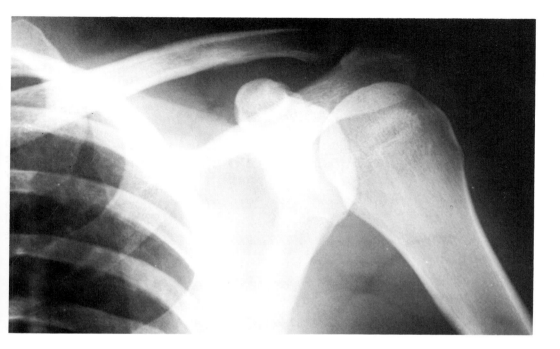

Fig 56 An X-ray of the shoulder joint.

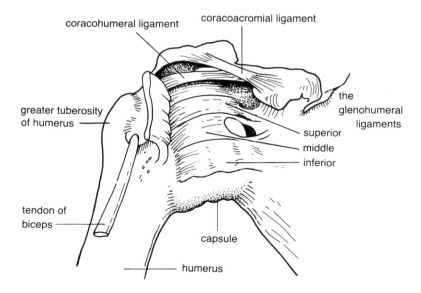

Fig 57 Anterior aspect of the right shoulder joint.

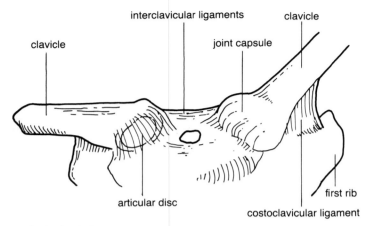

Fig 58   The sternoclavicular joints.

classed as a double-plane joint because a fibrocartilaginous disc lies within the articulation and divides the joint into two compartments (*see* Fig 58).

The Acromioclavicular Joint

This joint is a synovial-plane joint and is formed by the articulation of the lateral end of the clavicle with the acromion process of scapula. The capsule is reinforced by the acromioclavicular ligament. Other ligaments of importance here include the coracoclavicular ligament which runs from the underneath of the clavicle to the coracoid process of the scapula and the coracoacromial ligament which runs from the acromion process to the coracoid process (*see* Fig 59).

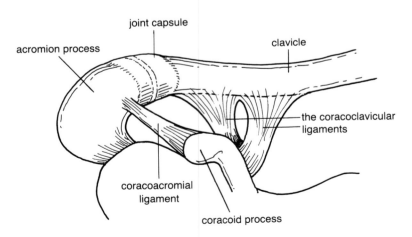

Fig 59   The acromioclavicular joint.

Strains of the Shoulder Muscles

Intrinsic strains of the shoulder muscles are infrequent but when they happen they are best treated according to the principles which apply to any other muscle injury of a similar nature.

Injury to the Acromioclavicular Joint

The acromioclavicular joint may be injured by a fall on to the shoulder in which, at the moment of impact, the acromion process is fixed, but the clavicle continues to move as a result of the player's momentum, thus causing the ligaments of the acromioclavicular joint to be sprained, partially torn or ruptured, according to the degree of force applied to the joint. The first-aid treatment for the sprain or first degree of injury will include the application of an ice-pack for the recommended period of time followed by strapping which should pass over the top of the shoulder and under the forearm with the elbow fixed at 90°. The arm is then rested in a broad arm-sling (*see* Fig 60).

With the second degree of injury the player will be unable to continue the game. Having once removed the player from the field an X-ray at hospital must be the first priority and the hospital staff will then decide on a treatment programme.

In the case of a rupture of the

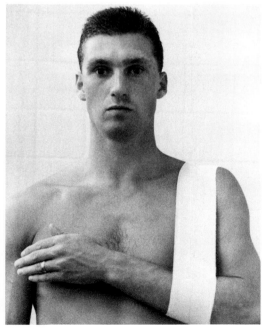

Fig 60   The support strapping for a sprain of the left acromioclavicular joint.

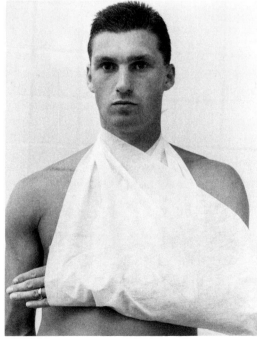

Fig 61   An arm-sling in position.

acromioclavicular ligaments the symptoms that the player initially displays will be very similar to those for a fracture, so the priorities on the field must first be to diagnose the severity of injury, the structures involved and then to immobilise the joint before transporting the player from the field and on to hospital for an X-ray examination.

DISLOCATION OF THE SHOULDER JOINT

Dislocation of the glenohumeral joint is a serious injury which presents few diagnostic problems – the symptoms are obvious. Firstly the player will be suffering excruciating pain and a complete loss of active function, nor will he be able to press his elbow into his side. He will also be supporting the elbow and forearm of the affected shoulder. When the shoulder is dislocated the head of the humerus separates from the glenoid cavity, producing considerable deformity. This deformity is shown clinically by the flattening over the upper part of the shoulder and may even be visible through the player's football shirt; if not, it will certainly be palpable.

The treatment on the field is to immobilise and support the affected arm, but in my experience the player himself will feel happier to hold his own arm rather than allow the immobilisation and support of triangular bandages. This decision is one for the practical situation, common sense being the guiding principle. You must immediately arrange for the player to be taken to hospital.

FRACTURES TO THE CLAVICLE

The causes of injury here can vary considerably since the clavicle can be fractured by a direct blow, a fall on an outstretched arm or a fall on to the point of the shoulder. The symptoms you will meet will include considerable pain, a gross loss of active function, localised swelling and a deformity may be detectable. The treatment required on the field is, once again, to immobilise the fracture with the use of a triangular bandage to form a sling. This method may be used if the player is able to walk from the field, but when the player is in shock, a stretcher is the safest means of transportation from the field. Having arrived at hospital an X-ray examination will be required to confirm the diagnosis.

10 Elbow Injuries

ANATOMICAL CONSIDERATION

The elbow is classed as a synovial hinge joint allowing flexion and extension to take place. The articulation (or movement) is between the trochlea and the capitulum on the lower end of the humerus with the trochlea notch on the ulna and the head of the radius. There is a capsule that surrounds the articular margins, and the synovial membrane is situated on its inner surface. The joint is stabilised by collateral ligaments – both medial and lateral – which have attachments to the epicondyle of the humerus. The medial ligament passes downwards to split into three bands along the medial aspect of the ulna to the coronoid process, the olecranon process and a connecting band between the two processes. The lateral ligament is attached to the annular ligament which surrounds the head of the radius.

The movements controlled by the elbow are flexion and extension, the range being determined by the volume of muscle on the anterior aspect of the arm and forearm.

FRACTURES

In football fractures of the elbow can occur to the olecranon process and the head of the radius. The cause of such an injury would normally be direct contact.

If you suspect a fracture following your initial examination, arrange to have the player transported to hospital. A broad arm-sling application is the best method of support until the player reaches hospital.

DISLOCATIONS

Dislocation of the elbow joint is an extremely serious injury. However, it is

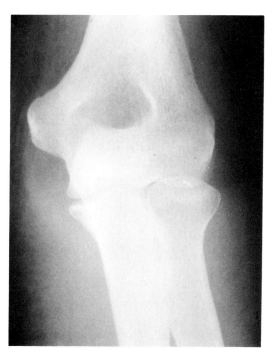

Fig 62 An X-ray of the elbow joint.

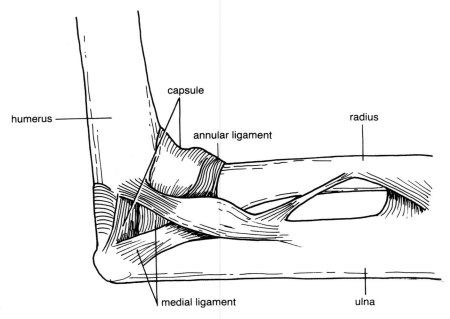

Fig 63   *Left elbow joint, medial view.*

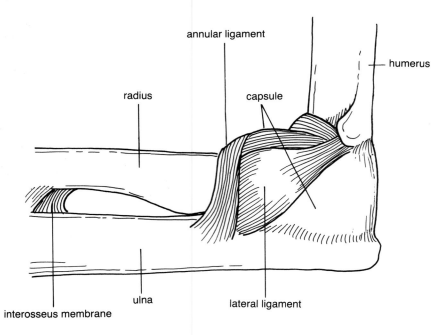

Fig 64   *Left elbow joint, lateral view.*

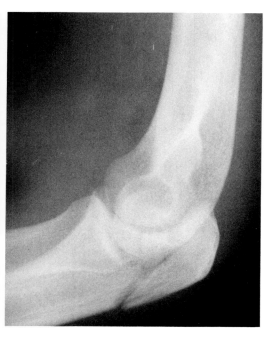

Fig 65 An X-ray showing a fracture of the olecranon process.

head of the radius and of the coronoid process of the ulna are also seen on X-ray examination. The major problem with a dislocated elbow is that the blood supply to the hand and arm may be severely affected by arterial spasm. If you suspect this, periodically check the radial (wrist) pulse and also the colour and temperature of the forearm and hand. The player should be transported from the field on a stretcher with the injured arm supported against his body by triangular bandages. He should then be taken by ambulance to hospital.

SPRAINS OF THE ELBOW JOINT

The ligaments that stabilise the elbow joint are occasionally sprained by the elbow being forced into extension. This produces an injury to the anterior attachments of the collateral ligaments. The symptoms include; pain, when the affected ligament is stressed, tenderness on palpation, swelling, and a limitation of function.

It is important to remember that *unlike* sprains in ligament tissue of a first or second degree in other joints, the elbow is *not* immobilised by a pressure bandage, but supported by a sling with the elbow rested at 90°.

easily diagnosed simply because of the immense pain the player will be suffering. The deformity can be considerable with the olecranon process of the ulna projecting backwards – obviously active movement is not possible. For the joint to become dislocated, the collateral ligaments need to have ruptured and in some extreme cases a fracture of the

11 Wrist and Finger Injuries

ANATOMICAL CONSIDERATIONS

The Wrist Joint

The wrist joint is formed by the inferior (or inner) surfaces of the radius and ulna and the scaphoid, lunate and triquetral bones. It is called a synovial condyloid joint because it allows flexion, extension, abduction (an outward movement) and adduction (an inward movement) to take place; rotation, however, does not take place at the wrist. The joint is strengthened by the medial ligament on its medial aspect which is attached to the ulna and to the triquetral bones. Laterally, the joint is strengthened by the lateral ligament which is attached to the radius and at its lower end to the scaphoid.

The Carpal and Carpometacarpal Joints

The carpal joints control the articulation of the eight carpal bones, which are arranged in two rows of four. The proximal or upper row which are situated closest to the radius and ulna are named scaphoid, lunate, triquetral and pisiform. The distal or lower row of bones are termed trapezium, trapezoid, capitate and hamate (*see* Fig 67).

The Carpometacarpal Joint of the Thumb

The articulation is between the trapezium and the base of the first metacarpal bone. It is classed as a saddle joint as the range of movements

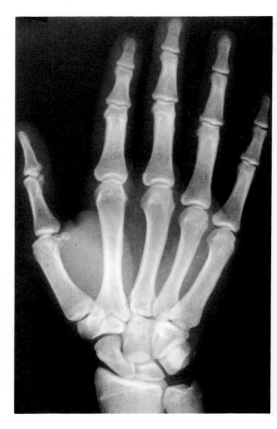

Fig 66   *An X-ray of the wrist and fingers.*

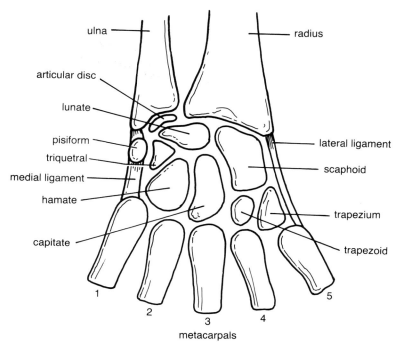

Fig 67   The bones of the wrist.

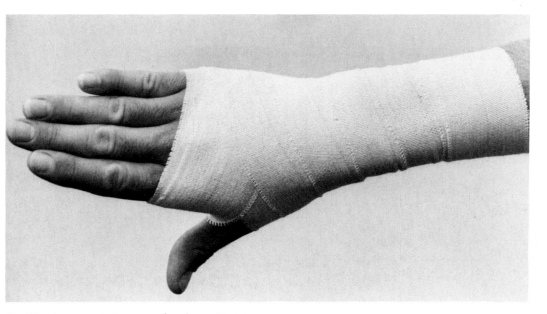

Fig 68   A support strapping for the wrist joint.

71

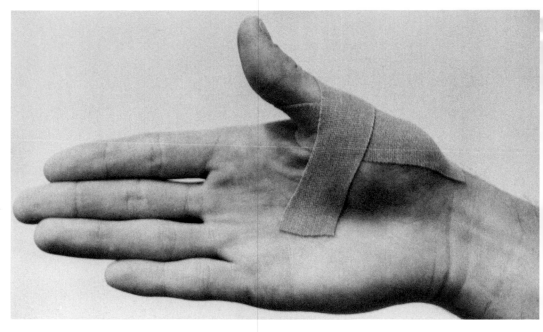

Fig 69   *A support tape for the first metacarpophalangeal joint.*

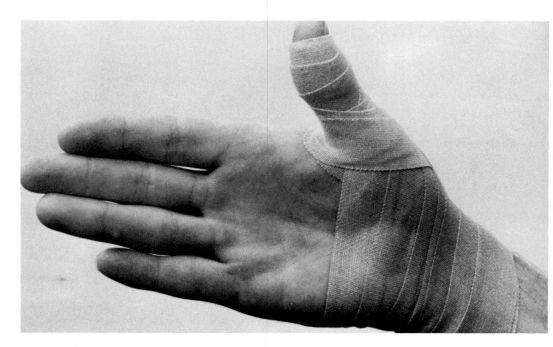

Fig 70   *The completed support strapping for the first metacarpophalangeal joint.*

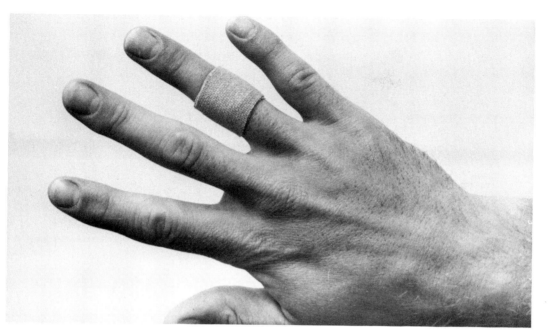

Fig 71   A support tape for a phalangeal joint injury.

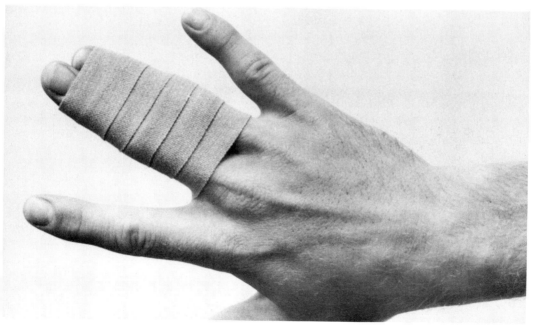

Fig 72   The completed support strapping for a phalangeal joint
injury.

are abduction, adduction (the inward and outward range), flexion and extension. The movement of the thumb being drawn across the palm of the hand is called apposition.

The Metacarpophalangeal Joints

The articulation is between the heads of the metacarpal bones and the bases of the proximal phalanges of each finger. These joints are termed synovial condyloid joints.

The Interphalangeal Joints

These are the joints of the fingers which have a mechanism of flexion and extension. They are stabilised by the collateral ligaments and are classed as synovial hinge joints.

INJURIES

Injuries to the wrist and fingers in soccer are infrequent. Players may from time to time suffer a sprain of the ligaments that stabilise the joint. The injury is usually caused by the wrist being forced backwards into extension when falling to the ground or, less commonly, by the ball being kicked very hard on to the hand, forcing the wrist into involuntary extension. This cause of injury, however, is more frequent amongst goalkeepers, their interphalangeal joints being stressed into hyperextension by the force of the ball.

The treatment in the initial stage of injury does not differ:

1. X-ray.
2. Ice.
3. Support and compression.
4. Rest.
5. Elevation.

The X-ray examination of a wrist or finger injury is of great importance if there is the slightest indication of a fracture. Falling on to an outstretched hand may produce a sprain, but if the weight distribution and speed of impact is great enough, a Colles fracture or a fracture of the scaphoid may occur. The Colles fracture is a break of the lower part of the radius and causes considerable pain, the so-called 'dinner-fork' deformity, lack of active movement and an immediate effusion. The first-aid treatment must be to apply a broad arm-sling and take the player immediately to hospital for an X-ray and specialist treatment. In the case of a scaphoid fracture there will be acute pain in the area of the affected bone (situated at the base of the thumb). The major symptoms to look for are that extension of the wrist is both limited and painful to perform, there may be localised swelling over the bones and most significantly, the player will be unable to grip firmly with the injured hand. An X-ray examination of course, is required to confirm the diagnosis.

Fractures of the scaphoid often take a long time to unite. Non-union is not uncommon and sometimes surgical interference (a bone graft or pinning) is necessary.

12 Spinal Injuries

ANATOMICAL CONSIDERATIONS

The spine consists of thirty-three vertebrae starting at the base of the skull and passing down to the pelvic region. The upper twenty-four are separate and mobile while the lower nine are fused to form the sacrum and coccyx. Of the higher section the upper seven vertebrae are termed cervical, the middle twelve are called the thoracic vertebrae and the lower five the lumbar. The joints between the vertebrae are cartilaginous and each contains an intervertebral disc situated between the bones. The function of this disc is to act as a shock absorber and assist joint movement. Each individual vertebral disc is attached to the anterior and posterior longitudinal ligaments, which also bind the bodies of the vertebrae together (see Fig 73).

The spinal cord passes down inside the spinal canal which lies behind the vertebral bodies extending from the base of the skull downwards to the first lumbar vertebra. The remaining part of the lumbar canal transmits nerve roots. As the cord descends it gives off thirty-one pairs of spinal nerves which emerge through the intervertebral foramina (holes in the bones of the spine) which are situated at the sides of each of the adjacent vertebrae. There are in all eight cervical, twelve thoracic, five lumbar, five sacral and one coccygeal pairs of spinal nerves. The peripheral nerves

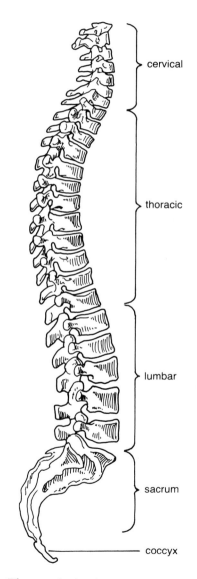

Fig 73 *The vertebral column.*

cervical

thoracic

lumbar

sacrum

coccyx

75

supply and relay both motor and sensory stimuli to and from the voluntary muscles, joints and skin. (It should be understood that the term 'lumbar', 'sacral', and 'coccygeal' when applied to the spinal cord do not correspond to those regions of the vertebral column similarly named.)

INJURIES

Injuries affecting the spinal region are fortunately infrequent in football; the last recorded fracture was received during the World Cup Finals in Spain in 1982. The incident occurred when the German goalkeeper Harald Schumacher collided with the French full back, Patrick Battiston during the semi-final between the two countries. Battiston received three fractured cervical vertebrae as a result of the collision and was taken from the pitch on a stretcher.

The FA Cup Final of 1956 was between Manchester City and Birmingham City. The Manchester team were leading 3–1 with just fifteen minutes remaining. Bert Trautmann, the Manchester City goalkeeper, threw himself bravely at the feet of Peter Murphy to deny the Birmingham forward a scoring opportunity. The resulting contact produced a fracture to a cervical vertebra and although obviously in great pain Trautmann continued until the final whistle was blown. A post-match X-ray examination revealed the fracture.

Management

The symptoms a player will display following an injury to his spine, whether the injury be a fracture or a prolapsed (slipped) disc, will be:

1. Pain, localised to the site of the injury.
2. Referred pain, radiated into the shoulder, arm (in the case of a lumbar spinal injury, the leg) or hand.
3. Pins and needles.
4. Numbness.
5. Weakness in the muscles of the region related to the level of the fracture.

The correct first-aid treatment on the field of play is to support the neck in a cervical collar before placing the injured player on the stretcher. The lifting of the casualty must be organised in advance to avoid any unnecessary movement. Transportation to hospital should be immediate – this is an emergency case.

13 Hip Injuries

ANATOMICAL CONSIDERATIONS

The articulation of the hip joint is between the hemispherical head of the femur and the cup-shaped acetabular cavity on the innominate bone. The joint is classed as a synovial ball and socket and is surrounded by a capsule which is reinforced by the iliofemoral ligament, the pubofemoral ligament and at the back by the ischiofemoral ligament (*see* Figs 75 and 76).

The movements that take place at the hip joint are: flexion (the thigh bending forward), this movement is limited by the hamstrings when the knee is extended; extension (the thigh pressing backwards), this movement is assisted by the hamstrings; abduction (moving the thigh outwards); adduction (moving the thigh inwards). Two rotational movements occur at the hip joint; the lateral rotation (the movement of the thigh turning outwards) and the medial rotation (the movement of the thigh turning inwards). Occasionally you will be presented with soft-tissue injuries in the region of the hip joint. The first-aid treatment for these injuries is identical to that for any other region of the body.

Case History

In 1973, at the height of his career, Bobby Kerr captained Sunderland FC to an FA Cup Final victory. After a long and distinguished career with the Roker Park club he joined Blackpool FC. During a third division game against Bury at Bloomfield Road, Bobby suffered a posterior hip dislocation. To my knowledge this is the only dislocation to the hip joint ever sustained in Assocation Football.

The incident occurred when Bobby chased a ball down the right side of midfield and on reaching the ball was tackled. The force of the tackle from the

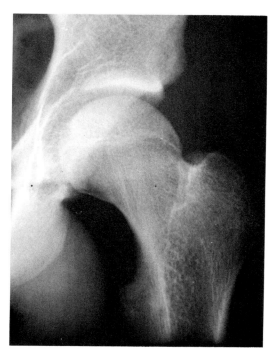

Fig 74   An X-ray of the hip joint.

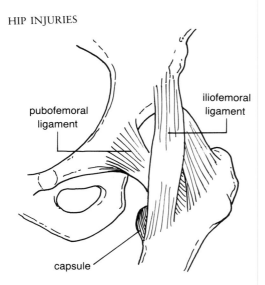

Fig 75   *Left hip joint, anterior aspect.*

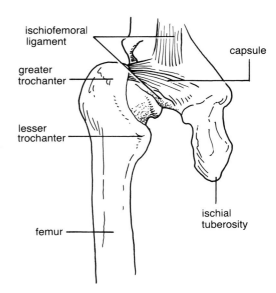

Fig 76   *Left hip joint, posterior aspect.*

front coincided with a blow into his back and the combination of forces brought about his hip dislocation. On reaching the player, it was clear he was suffering considerable pain, the affected leg was 'shortened' and internally rotated. He was resting his foot on top of the sound leg and a prominence of the greater trochanter of the femur was palpable (*see* Fig 78).

I immobilised the legs by using triangular bandages tied at intervals down the full length of the legs, so immobilising the injured limb and joint as much as was possible without moving the player. I then ensured that the stretcher was positioned at the player's feet so that he could be lifted and the stretcher slid underneath his body. The carrying of the stretcher had to be managed very carefully in order to prevent any unnecessary movement. He was then immediately transported by ambulance to hospital where he was treated by an orthopaedic specialist who supervised the X-ray, operative reduction (repositioning of the bones) and traction.

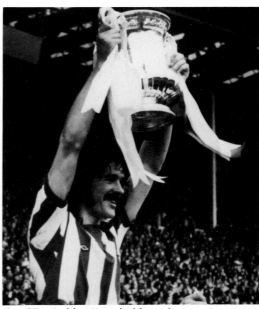

Fig 77   *Bobby Kerr holding the FA Cup in 1973. During the course of a game against Bury FC (when playing for Blackpool FC) he suffered a posterior hip dislocation – one of the most unusual injuries sustained in football. (Photo: Sunderland Echo.)*

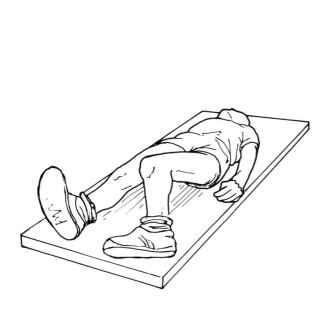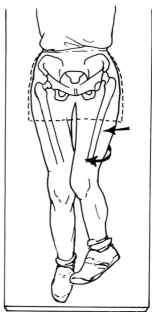

Fig 78 A diagrammatic interpretation of the position of a player who has suffered a dislocated hip. Note the 'shortened' leg and the internally rotated (adducted) thigh. The casualty is likely to be supporting the injured foot on top of his sound foot. You may also detect a lateral prominence of the greater trochanter of the femur.

The lesson to be learned from this situation is that on reaching a player on the field, you should use a process of elimination so far as diagnosis is concerned; consider the most serious injury first and eliminate the severe possibilities quickly and methodically in your mind. Having reached a diagnosis, you may then treat accordingly. Never pre-diagnose and never underestimate any situation.

14 Abdominal Injuries

ANATOMICAL CONSIDERATIONS

The abdominal region passes up from the pelvic region to the diaphragm. The broad function of this area is to support and protect the contents of the abdomen; it is a continuation of the trunk, helping to support the body-weight in the region of the back since the lumbar spine gives a great deal of skeletal support, the muscular support being provided by a very strong structure of muscles (*see* Fig 79). Extending forwards from the posterior (back) to the anterior (front) area are the abdominal muscles. This muscle-path converges into the fascia in the front which then splits to include the rectus abdomini muscles (*see* Fig 80).

The lower ribs protect the upper part of the abdominal cavity and cover the major portion of the liver, spleen and, to a lesser extent, the kidneys (*see* Fig 81). In the front the two recti muscles pass from the lower ribs to the pubis, helping to provide an erect posture and assisting the anterior spinal muscles in performing forward flexion (*see* Fig 82).

INJURIES TO THE ABDOMINAL WALL

Contusions

A contusion is caused by a direct blow producing the following symptoms of localised pain – tenderness to the touch and a degree of spasm. An ice-pack should be applied to the affected area for a period of fifteen minutes followed by a rest period of twenty-four hours. The symptoms should subside very quickly following this type and degree of injury.

Strains

A strain is produced either by overuse or by a sudden movement which stretches or slightly tears a few fibres of the abdominal muscle. Having reached a diagnosis, once again the principles of ice and rest should be applied, followed by an appointment for physiotherapy.

Hernias

If a player experiences persistent pain in the abdominal region when striking a football, sprinting or following endurance runs, he must be referred to a doctor. If coughing and sneezing are painful – particularly so in the evening or after standing all day – these, too, are symptoms associated with a hernia. A consultation with either the club doctor or the player's own general practitioner is required.

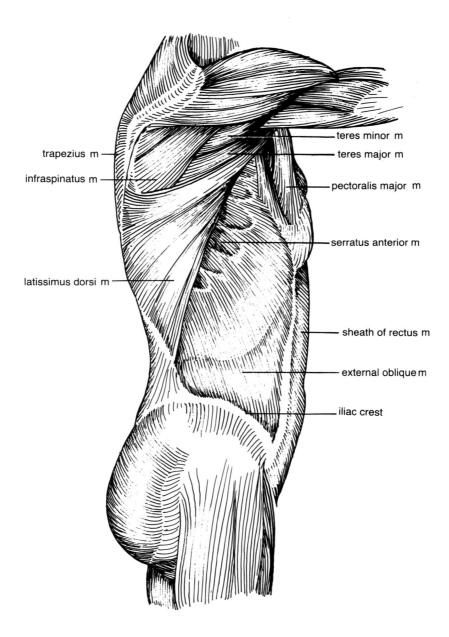

trapezius m

infraspinatus m

latissimus dorsi m

teres minor m

teres major m

pectoralis major m

serratus anterior m

sheath of rectus m

external oblique m

iliac crest

Fig 79   A lateral view of the abdominal area showing the interdigitation of the abdominal muscles with the muscles of the back, shoulder and chest at the top, and the attachment to the iliac crest below.

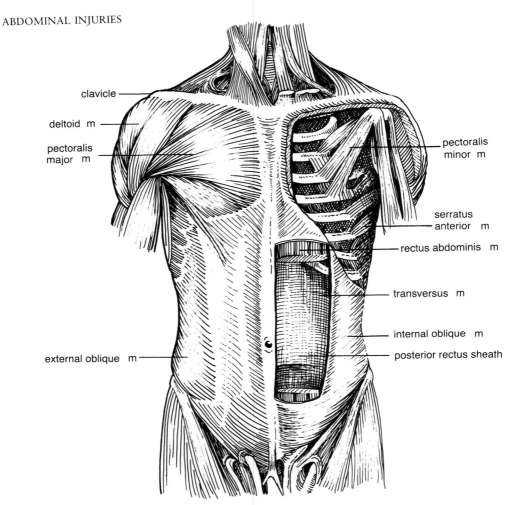

Fig 80 Note the intimate relationship between the muscles of the chest and abdomen.

INJURY TO THE ABDOMINAL CONTENT

Fortunately injury to the abdominal content in soccer is infrequent. From time to time players suffer direct blows to this region, but the majority of injuries are muscular complaints. If one of your players does receive a direct blow to the abdominal region during a game you must, of course, diagnose the injury and give initial treatment. The answers to the following questions should be considered when forming your diagnosis:

1. Is the injury the result of a direct blow?
2. What was it that hit the player? Was it the ball? Was it kicked from close range into the abdominal region? Was the player elbowed in the side or

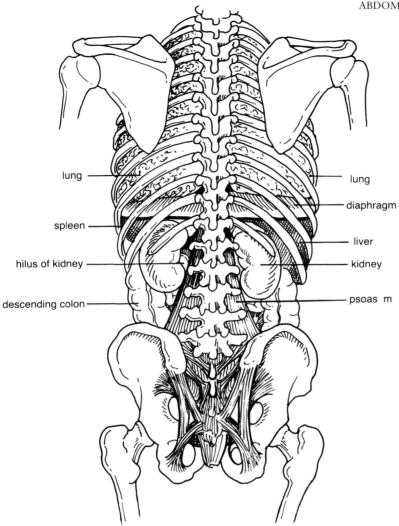

lung

lung

diaphragm

spleen

liver

hilus of kidney

kidney

descending colon

psoas m

Fig 81 A posterior view to show the position of the spleen on the left.
Note the position of the kidneys and the liver on the right.

kicked in the back? Was an opponent's knee involved in the incident?
3.   What was the position of the player's body at the time of the blow?
4.   Were the player's muscles tense at the time of contact or was he relaxed and off-guard?
5.   Where is the site of the injury? Is it in the back, sides or front of the abdominal region? Where is the pain ? Is it abdominal, or over the liver, kidneys or spleen?
6.   What symptoms is the player displaying? These might include nausea, vomiting, pallor, a cold and clammy skin or other signs of shock.

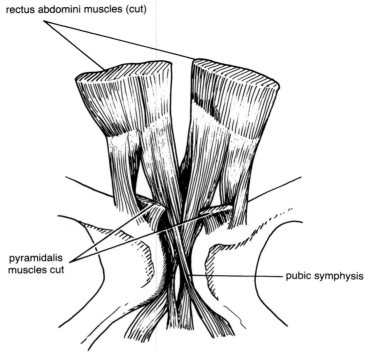

rectus abdomini muscles (cut)

pyramidalis
muscles cut

pubic symphysis

Fig 82   The insertion of the rectus abdomini muscles into the pubic region.

Other Symptoms and Initial Treatment

A player who has received a blow to the stomach will probably be struggling for breath, as well as having considerable pain and cramp in the abdomen. Other possible symptoms include a rapid pulse, dizziness and fainting, all of which are caused by blood loss through internal bleeding. If the symptoms subside quickly he may feel sufficiently recovered to continue the game, but if there is any doubt the player should be removed from the field and examined first by yourself and then – if necessary – by a doctor. If the injury is at all severe, the casualty must be taken from the pitch on a stretcher and transported to hospital by ambulance. Be ready to tell the doctor of the history of the injury and any observations you may have made.

INJURY TO THE KIDNEY

The most common kidney injury is the contusion. This is normally the result of a blow from a knee, elbow, boot or even the ball with the shock penetrating the muscles and being transmitted to the kidney. The symptoms of this injury are localised pain and the presence of blood in the urine. A player with these symptoms should be taken immediately to hospital for examination by a doctor.

84

OTHER INJURIES OF THE ABDOMEN

Injuries to the spleen are most unusual in soccer but when they occur, they are always caused by a direct blow. The symptoms are due entirely to internal bleeding (dizziness, feeling faint and a rapid pulse). Immediate transportation to hospital should be arranged – this is an emergency case. Injuries to the liver, pancreas, bladder and the intestinal tract are extremely uncommon in soccer. Contusion of the abdominal wall may well cause some contusion to the underlying stomach or intestines, but these organs are pliable and usually give with the blow sufficiently so that they are not damaged when pressed between the abdominal wall and the spine. The unusual eventuality of a direct blow so severe as to rupture the bowel will give immediate and serious symptoms: abdominal pain; tenderness; spasm; nausea; vomiting.

In some cases of injury to the abdominal contents the symptoms may develop gradually and some time after the injury has occurred, possibly as much as a number of hours after the game. It is of the utmost importance to inform the player's family that if any symptoms reappear he should be immediately taken to the nearest hospital. This instruction must be given after a post-match examination has been carried out by a doctor. If any blood can be seen in the player's urine following an abdominal injury, you must insist that he is taken to hospital for specialist examination and treatment.

Appendix 1

CONTENTS OF THE TRAINER'S BAG

The Field Bag

To be able to treat injuries on the field of play a number of medical items are required. The following is a list of the equipment that I myself take in my field bag for the first-aid treatment of injuries:

1. A bottle of water, useful when dealing with contusions or abrasions.

2. A bottle of Cetavlon 1%, a valuable cleaning agent.
3. A pain-relieving spray. This method of first-aid treatment is a local anaesthetic which should be applied only after careful examination and accurate diagnosis.
4. A jar of Vaseline or white petroleum jelly.
5. Elastoplast strapping of width 7.5 cm (3in).
6. Elastoplast strapping of width 5cm (2in).

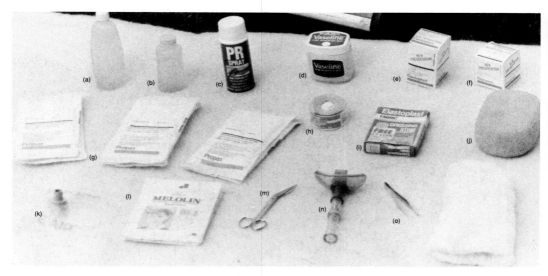

Fig 83 The contents of the trainer's bag: (a) bottle of water (b) Cetavlon 1% (c) pain-relief spray (d) Vaseline (e) elastoplast strapping, width 7.5cm (3in) (f) elastoplast strapping, width 5cm (2in) (g) triangular bandages (h) elastoplast strapping, width 2.5cm (1in) (i) dressing strip, width 7.5cm (3in) (j) sponge (k) airway (l) sterile dressings (m) scissors (n) Brook airway (o) tweezers.

7. Triangular bandages, used for immobilising fractures or dislocations. I tend to carry six in my bag.
8. Adhesive tape of width 2.5cm (1in).
9. Dressing strip of width 7.5cm (3in).
10. Sponge, this has many practical uses; keep it clean and in a separate bag.
11. A Johnson & Johnson resuscitator.
12. Melolin sterile dressings, for use when treating an open wound.
13. Scissors. Choose scissors with bevelled ends in order to avoid the risk of a sharp point catching the skin when cutting tape or clothing.
14. A Brook airway.
15. Tweezers.
16. Cotton wool.

All these items should be small so that they will fit into your field bag. Do not overload, and arrange the contents for easy availability.

Other Equipment

Ensure you have available and close to the field a good quality stretcher and blankets. Splints and an ordinary bucket for cold water should also be to hand. In addition to the field bag a medical case, more comprehensively stocked than the field bag, should be provided. This can be placed with the stretcher, blankets, bucket and splints within easy reach of the field of play.

1. Inflatable splints.
2. Ice-packs.
3. Crêpe bandages width 15cm (6in).
4. Hospital-quality cotton wool.
5. Tinaderm powder for athlete's foot.
6. Cicatrin powder 50g.
7. Spenco 'second skin'.
8. Tubigrip size C and G.
9. Paracetamol BP 500mg.
10. Surgical felt.

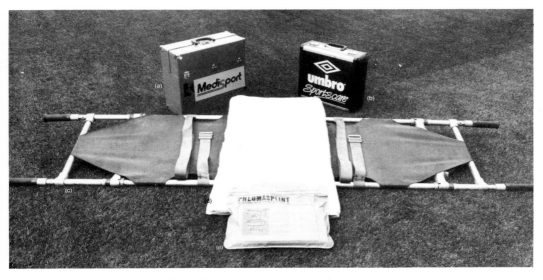

Fig 84   The equipment that should be within easy reach of the field of play: (a) medical case (b) field bag (c) stretcher (d) blankets (e) splints.

11. Scissors (four pairs).
12. Thermometer.
13. Razor.
14. Liniment.
15. Cetavlon 1%.
16. Elastoplast adhesive strapping, the following widths: 2.5cm (1in); 5cm (2in); 7.5cm (3in).
17. Tubifoam.
18. Dressings: melolin, 10×10cm (4in×4in); fucidin gauze dressings, 10×10cm (4in×4in).
19. Kidney-shaped dish.
20. A jar of white petroleum jelly.
21. (Anti-catarrh) smelling salts.
22. Algipan rub.
23. Vick rub.
24. Cotton bandage of width 7.5cm (3in).
25. Dumb-bell sutures.
26. A bottle of kaolin and morphine.
27. Zinc oxide tape of width 2.5cm (1in).
28. Optrex solution and eye-bath.
29. A collapsible pair of crutches.
30. Unichem sterile dressing packs.

Appendix 2

THE POST-INJURY FITNESS TEST

Two tests should be undertaken before a player can be correctly passed as fit to play soccer. Firstly, he must be subjected to a clinical examination and then, having satisfied the examiner, he must be given a functional test.

Clinical Testing

In the case of leg, arm and shoulder injuries these tests should be made in comparison to the sound limb:

1. There should be no pain on palpation.
2. There should be a full range of active and passive movement of the joint or joints involved.
3. There should be equal and full extensibility of the muscle groups affected.
4. A series of 'resisted movements' of muscles acting on the affected joints should be carried out.
5. Stress testing of the injured ligaments should also be conducted.

Functional Testing

Following a thorough warm-up it is important to use a test which involves a series of sprints, checks and turns (shuttle-running). The player must also be able to manipulate the ball with controlling techniques using various parts of the body – for example, the chest, thighs and both feet. Passing the ball at gradually increasing distances with the necessary change of technique should form a part of the fitness test, as should driving, chipping and shooting. Other skills to incorporate in the test might include heading the ball from a standing position and then jumping to head the ball or small-sided games arranged in a grid so that the emphasis is on tackling.

If the player recovering from injury is a goalkeeper, the test will, of course, need to be modified. A variety of different skills need to be tested, but the following should be included as a minimum: sprinting; jumping and diving (to collect the ball from crosses and shots); throwing; volleying and half-volleying the ball and taking goal-kicks.

You should devise variations on these themes, incorporating a number of different skills, but you must always ensure that the outcome of a successful test is that both you *and* the player feel confident and satisfied with his performance and fitness. Two other points to remember: if you have any doubts about a player's fitness, he should not take the field; and any player who has received a head injury must not return to playing or competitive training until he has been passed fit to do so by a doctor.

Glossary

Abdomen The lower part of the trunk. The upper part is the chest.

Acetabulum The cup-shaped socket of the pelvis for the head of the femur.

Acromion The part of the scapula (shoulder-blade) forming the tip of the shoulder.

Adhesion The uniting of structures which should normally be separate.

Arteriole A small artery.

Artery The blood vessel taking blood from the heart to the rest of the body.

Articular Of or related to a joint.

Aspiration The withdrawal of fluid from a joint.

Athlete's foot A term applied to a fungal skin eruption on the foot, usually between the toes.

Blood The fluid which circulates through the arteries, capillaries and veins, exchanging vital fluids and gases with the bodily tissues.

Bones These form the framework upon which the rest of the body is built. Fractures are a very common type of soccer injury.

Bursa The natural hollow in fibrous tissue, lined by smooth cells and containing a little fluid. They help make the movement of the joint smooth.

Bursitis The inflammation of a bursa or of bursae.

Callus The new bone tissue which forms around fractures.

Capillary A minute blood vessel between the ends of the arteries and the beginning of the veins.

Cell A microscopic particle of which all tissue is made.

Cellulitis The inflammation of cellular tissue.

Clavicle Another name for the collarbone.

Coagulation The process in which bleeding is staunched in the body.

Coccyx The name of the lower end of the spinal column.

Collagen The major structural component in the body; it is a protein found in bones, tendons and elsewhere.

Colles fracture A fracture of the lower end of the radius.

Condyle A rounded prominence at the end of the bone.

Contusion A bruise.

Costal Pertaining to the ribs.

Cramp A painful spasmodic contraction of a muscle or muscles.

Crepitus A grating sound of a joint experienced after a fracture and in arthritic joints.

Dislocation An injury to a joint such that the end of adjacent bones are forced out of connection with one another.

Effusion Swelling.

Epiphysis The spongy extremity of a bone, which in a young person is connected with the shaft of the bone by a plate of cartilage – this disappears in adulthood.

Extension The extended position of a joint (as opposed to flexion).

Fascia The thin sheet of fibrous tissues

which encloses and connects the muscles.

Femur   The thigh-bone.

Fibrous tissue   One of the most abundant tissues throughout the body, the fibres usually made up of collagen.

Fibula   The slender bone on the outer side of the lower leg.

Flexion   The term for the bending of joints (the opposite of extension).

Fractures   Fractures are breaches in the structure of bones caused either by external force or by stress.

Gastrocnemius   The muscle that forms the bulk of the calf.

Glenoid   The name of the cavity on the shoulder-blade into which the humerus fits.

Greenstick Fracture   A fracture which occurs in children; the long bones are incompletely fractured, thus showing on X-ray examination as a 'bending' of the bone rather than a complete break.

Haemarthrosis   Bleeding into, or the presence of blood in, a joint.

Haematoma   A collection of blood forming a swelling.

Haemoglobin   The pigment which produces the red colour of blood and which is used in 'transporting' oxygen around the body.

Haemorrhage   This means the escape of blood from the vessels which naturally contain it.

Haemothorax   An effusion of blood into the pleural cavity.

Hernia   The protrusion of any organ or part of an organ into or through the wall of the cavity which contains it.

Humerus   The bone of the upper arm.

Inflammation   This may be defined as the reaction of the tissues to any injury.

Joint   The meeting place between different parts of the skeleton.

Ligament   A strong band of fibrous tissue which serves to stabilise joints. In some cases the ligament may be cord-like, in others flattened bands. Most joints are surrounded by a fibrous, capsular ligament.

March fracture   A form of stress fracture usually occurring in the second metatarsal bone.

Meniscectomy   The surgical removal of cartilage.

Metacarpal   One of five long bones in the hand between the carpal bones at the wrist and the phalanges of the fingers.

Metatarsal   One of five bones in the foot which correspond to the metacarpal bones of the hand.

Orthopaedics   The branch of medicine dealing with correction of deformities of bones and mucles.

Ossification   The growth and formation of bone.

Osteitis   Inflammation of the bone substance.

Osteochondritis   Inflammation of both bone and cartilage.

Osteomyelitis   Inflammation of the marrow of the bone.

Patella   The technical name for the knee-cap.

Physiotherapy   Treatment of injury using massage and exercise rather than drugs.

Plasma   The fluid constituent of the blood.

Platelet   A very small, roughly spherical body in the blood which plays an important part in the process of blood coagulation.

Pleural cavity   The lungs are enveloped in the pleural membrane in such a way that one layer of the membrane adheres closely to the lungs, whilst the other layer lines the inner surface of the chest.

These two layers form a closed cavity: the pleural cavity.

Quadriceps The muscle group at the front and sides of the thigh.

Radius The outer of the two bones in the forearm.

Ribs Twelve pairs of ribs enclose the cavity of the chest.

Rupture A term used for a hernia or complete severance of a structure in the body.

Scapula The technical name for the shoulder-blade.

Sprain A first-degree injury to a ligament.

Spring ligament The most important ligament in the foot, it supports the head of the talus, which carries the weight of the body. It is also called the calcaneonavicular ligament.

Sternum The technical name for the breastbone.

Strain A first-degree injury to a muscle.

Synovitis Inflammation of the membrane lining of a joint.

Tendon The cord-like structure that attaches the end of a muscle to bone or other structures upon which the muscle acts when it contracts.

Tenosynovitis Inflammation of a tendon.

Thorax The technical name for the chest.

Tibia The technical name for the shin-bone.

Tinea The technical name for ring worm.

Trauma The term used to indicate the tissue reaction to wounds and injuries.

Trochlear notch The articular surface of the ulna within the elbow joint.

Ulna The name of the inner of the two bones of the forearm.

Valgus Bending of the knees inwards, 'knock-kneed'.

Varus The bow-legged position.

Vein A vessel which carries blood to the heart after it has circulated through the tissues of the body.

Verruca (The Latin term for) a wart.

Useful Addresses

The following manufacturers may be contacted directly for further details regarding their products. Obviously, this list is by no means exhaustive.

BDF Medical Ltd
Yeoman's Drive
Blakelands
Milton Keynes
Buckinghamshire MK14 5LS

Tapes and strappings of varying sizes

Cuxson, Gerrard & Company Ltd
Oldbury
Warley
West Midlands B69 3BB

Fully equipped medical cases

Footman & Company Ltd
Grove Mill
475–479 London Road
Mitcham
Surrey CR4 4YP

Most chiropody products

Johnson & Johnson Patient Care Ltd
Coronation Road
Ascot
Berkshire SL5 9SY

Life aid resuscitators

Leo Laboratories Ltd
Longwick Road
Princes Risborough
Aylesbury
Buckinghamshire HP17 9RR

Fucidin Intertulle sterile gauze dressings

Medisport International Ltd
Jackson Close
Grove Road
Drayton
Portsmouth PO6 1UR

Fully equipped medical cases

The National Physiotherapy Service (and) Milas Ltd The Manor House Squires Hill Rothwell Northamptonshire	Elasticated adhesive tapes, zinc oxide tapes, adhesive foam, adhesive felt
Robinson's of Chesterfield Ltd Wheat Bridge Chesterfield Derbyshire S40 2AD	White surgical felt, cotton wool
Seton Products Ltd Tubiton House Oldham Lancashire OL1 3HS	Tubigrips, dumb-bell sutures, tubipads, tubifoams
Sportsystems (Medical) Ltd 13 Western Road Industrial Estate Stratford-upon-Avon Warwickshire CV37 0AH	Fully equipped medical cases
Squibb Surgicare Ltd Squibb House 141–149 Staines Road Hounslow Middlesex TW3 3JA	Granuflex hydroactive dressings
Thornton & Ross Ltd Linthwaite Laboratories Huddersfield West Yorkshire HD7 5QH	White petroleum jelly
Unichem Ltd Unichem House Cox's Lane Chessington Surrey KT9 1SN	Sterile dressing packs

Index